# A Critical Evaluation of Alternatives to Acute Ocular Irritation Testing

John M. Frazier, Ph.D.
Shayne C. Gad, Ph.D.
Alan M. Goldberg, Ph.D.
James P. McCulley, M.D.

*with special assistance in the
preparation of Chapter 5*

Dale R. Meyer, Ph.D.

Mary Ann Liebert, Inc. publishers

ALTERNATIVE METHODS IN TOXICOLOGY SERIES

Volume 1
Product Safety Evaluation

Volume 2
Acute Toxicity Testing: Alternative Approaches

Volume 3
*In Vitro* Methods in Toxicology

Volume 4
A Critical Evaluation of Alternatives to Acute Ocular Irritation Testing

Volume 5   (*in press*)
*In Vitro* Toxicology: Approaches to Validation

Copyright © 1987 by Mary Ann Liebert, Inc., Publishers, 1651 Third Avenue, New York, NY 10128

ISBN: 0-913-113-09-3

Printed in the United States of America

This volume was fully supported by a grant from Bausch & Lomb. We acknowledge their foresight, encouragement, and willingness to help establish a unique forum for evaluating work in progress. We sincerely appreciate their participation in this effort.

# Preface

The Center was approached by Bausch & Lomb to develop a project which would make a meaningful contribution to the advancement of *in vitro* alternatives to the Draize Eye Test. In a discussion with Bausch & Lomb, I suggested that we approach several individuals to write a draft monograph which would review the history and current status of eye irritancy testing; develop an understanding of the mechanistic basis of eye irritation; and review the currently suggested *in vitro* alternatives to eye irritancy testing. Further, this monograph would be distributed in draft form to those whose assays were being reviewed, but would be limited to about 50 individuals. It was also suggested that those that were invited to review the manuscript would participate in a one-day meeting where their comments would be heard by the authors, after which the monograph would be completed, with the sections on recommendations and summaries being written after the meeting. As a result, the recommendations presented are derived from the monograph and the workshop discussion.

In addition, four members of the Center's Advisory Board, Drs. Andrew Rowan, Robert Scala, David Maurice and John Strandberg, were asked to reexamine the final draft of the manuscript for its accuracy and completeness.

Drs. McCulley, Gad, Frazier, and I met several times during the preparation of the book and for its final completion. Additionally, Dr. Dale Meyer was largely responsible for the writing of Chapter 5, and for this I am most appreciative.

I would like to acknowledge the understanding and help of the participants (list follows). They contributed by providing us with both their published and unpublished materials. They provided us with written commentary on the draft document, making the final review comprehensive, and by participating openly at the meeting with critical, carefully thought-out-commentaries that acted as the backbone for discussion and understanding.

I would like to acknowledge most sincerely the dedicated and hard work of the authors. They were comprehensive in their review, met a timetable that bordered on the unrealistic, and worked with a sense of collaboration that made the task not only scientifically rewarding but fun. I anticipate that the approaches developed for this monograph will be useful for other aspects of our work and for those in other fields.

I would like to express my sincere appreciation for the organization, editing, prodding, and help provided by my Administrative Assistant, Marilyn Principe. She was always there to make sure that all progressed as planned and to support the authors and participants.

This volume does not mark the end of the process but the beginning. If such a workshop were held a year earlier there would have been inadequate information to review, and if postponed until a later date we would have missed the opportunity for critical peer evaluation at this early stage. I recognize that there will be many who will be disappointed in that we did not recommend a final test or battery. Scientifically this is not yet possible. We have, however, taken the next step toward developing acceptable *in vitro* methods to replace eye-irritancy testing in animals.

*Alan M. Goldberg*

# Contents

Preface                                                                           vii

Contributing Authors                                                               xi

Participants                                                                      xiii

**1**    Summary and Recommendations                                       1

**2**    Historical Perspective on Eye Irritation Testing                  5

**3**    Current *In Vivo* Testing Protocols, Procedures, and Practices    9

**4**    Adequacy of Current *In Vivo* Methods                            21

**5**    Potential Approaches for the Development of *In Vitro* Alternatives   31
     to Eye Irritancy Tests
     A.  Morphology                                             32
     B.  Cellular Toxicity                                      34
     C.  Cell and Tissue Physiology                             40
     D.  Inflammation/Immunity                                  41
     E.  Recovery/Repair                                        44

**6**    Critical Evaluation of Alternative Tests                         45
     A.  Introduction                                           45
     B.  Criteria for Test Evaluation                           47
     C.  Test Protocols                                         49

**7**    Validation                                                      113

   References                                                            119

# Contributing Authors

**John M. Frazier, Ph.D.**
Associate Professor of Environmental Health Sciences, The Johns Hopkins University School of Hygiene and Public Health, and Associate Director, The Johns Hopkins Center for Alternatives to Animal Testing, 615 North Wolfe Street, Baltimore, MD 21205

**Shayne C. Gad, Ph.D.**
Director of Toxicology, G.D. Searle & Co., 4901 Searle Parkway, Skokie, IL 60077

**Alan M. Goldberg, Ph.D.**
Director, The Johns Hopkins Center for Alternatives to Animal Testing, Professor of Environmental Health Sciences, and Associate Dean for Research, The Johns Hopkins University School of Hygiene and Public Health, 615 North Wolfe Street, Baltimore, MD 21205

**James P. McCulley, M.D.**
David Bruton, Jr. Professor and Chairman, Department of Ophthalmology, Southwestern Medical School, University of Texas Health Science Center at Dallas, 5323 Harry Hines Boulevard, Dallas, TX 75235

**Dale R. Meyer, Ph.D.**
Department of Ophthalmology, Southwestern Medical School, The University of Texas Health Science Center at Dallas, 5323 Harry Hines Boulevard, Dallas, TX 75235

# Participants

**Mario R. Angi, M.D.**
University of Padova, Italy

**Bradford Arthur**
Lilly Research Laboratories, Greenfield, IN

**Melvin W. Balk, D.V.M.**
Charles River Laboratories, Wilmington, MA

**Bryan Ballantyne, M.D., D.Sc., Ph.D.**
Charleston, WV

**Michael Balls, M.A., D.Phil.**
FRAME, United Kingdom

**Antonio Bettero, M.D.**
University of Padova, Italy

**Keith A. Booman, Ph.D.**
The Soap and Detergent Association, New York, NY

**Ellen Borenfreund, Ph.D.**
Laboratory Animal Research Center, Rockefeller University, New York, NY

**Carlo A. Benassi**
University of Padova, Italy

**Mildred G. Broome, Ph.D.**
Arthur D. Little, Inc., Cambridge, MA

**Kwan Y. Chan, Ph.D.**
University of Washington, Seattle, WA

**Vincent A. DeLeo, M.D.**
Columbia University, New York, NY

**Arno Driedger, Ph.D.**
Amway Corp., Ada, MI

**Robert Drotman**
Frito-Lay, Inc., Irving, TX

**Norman H. Dubin, Ph.D.**
The Johns Hopkins University, Baltimore, MD

**Stephen A. Elbert, Ph.D.**
Amoco Corp., Chicago, IL

**Salwa A. Elgebaly, Ph.D.**
University of Connecticut, Farmington, CT

**Kurt Enslein, Ph.D.**
Health Designs Inc., Rochester, NY

**Jeffrey Everitt, Ph.D.**
Chemical Industry Institute of Toxicology, Research Triangle Park, NC

**Larry L. Ewing, Ph.D.**
The Johns Hopkins University, Baltimore, MD

**Gary Flamm, Ph.D.**
United States Food and Drug Administration, Washington, DC

**John M. Frazier, Ph.D.**
The Johns Hopkins University, Baltimore, MD

**Shayne C. Gad, Ph.D.**
G.D. Searle and Co., Skokie, IL

**Alan M. Goldberg, Ph.D.**
The Johns Hopkins University, Baltimore, MD

**Virginia C. Gordon, Ph.D.**
National Testing Corp., Carson, CA

**Gareth M. Green, M.D.**
The Johns Hopkins University, Baltimore, MD

**Yale Gressel, Ph.D.**
Avon Products, Inc., Suffern, NY

**John F. Griffith, Ph.D.**
The Procter & Gamble Co., Cincinnati, OH

**Sharon Hainsworth**
Bausch & Lomb, Rochester, NY

**Ralph J. Helmsen, Ph.D.**
National Institutes of Health, Bethesda, MD

**Edward M. Jackson, Ph.D.**
Noxell Corp., Hunt Valley, MD

**Franklin T. Jepson**
Bausch & Lomb, Rochester, NY

**Marcia M. Jumblatt, M.A.**
Eye Research Institute, Boston, MA

**Barbara M. Kelley**
Bausch & Lomb, Rochester, NY

**Gerald L. Kennedy**
E.I. duPont de Nemours & Co., Haskell Laboratory for Toxicology and Industrial Medicine, Newark, DE

**Herman B.W.M. Koeter, Ph.D.**
TNO-CIVO Institutes, The Netherlands

**Paul Kotin, M.D.**
University of Colorado, Denver, CO

**Patricia L. Lang, Ph.D.**
Consultant to Charles River Labs, Wilmington, MA

**Joseph Leighton, M.D.**
The Medical College of Pennsylvania, Philadelphia, PA

**Niels P. Luepke, Ph.D.**
University of Muenster, Federal Republic of Germany

**Francis Marzulli, Ph.D.**
National Research Council, Rockville, MD

**David Maurice, Ph.D.**
Stanford University Medical Center, Stanford, CA

**James P. McCulley, M.D.**
The University of Texas Health Science Center at Dallas, Dallas, TX

**James McNerney, M.P.H.**
The Cosmetic, Toiletry and Fragrance Association, Inc., Washington, DC

**Dale R. Meyer, Ph.D.**
The University of Texas Health Science Center at Dallas, Dallas, TX

**Mary Mowrey-McKee, Ph.D.**
Bausch & Lomb, Rochester, NY

**Jerry Y. Niederkorn, Ph.D.**
The University of Texas Health Science Center at Dallas, Dallas, TX

**Arthur H. Neufeld, Ph.D.**
Eye Research Institute, Boston, MA

**Gerald A. Nixon**
The Procter & Gamble Co., Cincinnati, OH

**Helen North-Root, Ph.D.**
Armour-Dial, Inc., Scottsdale, AZ

**William E. Parish, Ph.D.**
Unilever Research, London, United Kingdom

**Samuel P. Phelan**
Taconic, Inc., Germantown NY

**Christoph A. Reinhardt, Ph.D.**
University of Zurich, Switzerland

**Michael Rosen**
Lever Bros., NY

**Geoffrey Rose, Ph.D.**
Shell Development Co., United Kingdom

**Andrew N. Rowan, D.Phil.**
Tufts University, Boston, MA

**Michael C. Scaife, Ph.D.**
Johnson & Johnson Ltd., United Kingdom

**Robert Scala, Ph.D.**
Exxon Corp., East Millstone, NJ

**John A. Shadduck, D.V.M., Ph.D.**
University of Illinois at Urbana-Champaign, Urbana, IL

**Robert W. Shimizu, Ph.D.**
Allergan, Irvine, CA

**Charles Shopsis, Ph.D.**
Laboratory Animal Research Center, Rockefeller University, New York, NY

**Henry Spira**
Coalition to Abolish Draize, New York, NY

**Dennis M. Stark, D.V.M., Ph.D.**
Laboratory Animal Research Center, Rockefeller University, New York, NY

**John D. Strandberg, D.V.M., Ph.D.**
The Johns Hopkins University, Baltimore, MD

**Ruy Tchao, Ph.D.**
Medical College of Pennsylvania, Philadelphia, PA

**Alexander G. Vongries, Ph.D.**
Colgate-Palmolive Co., Piscataway, NJ

**Patricia Williams, Ph.D.**
Bristol-Myers Co., Syracuse, NY

# Chapter 1

# Summary and Recommendations

This monograph was developed in order to examine the current proposed and/or suggested alternatives to rabbit eye irritancy testing. During the last five years, there has been an effort to develop new methods which would serve as alternatives to rabbit eye irritancy testing. It is the intent of this monograph to examine the appropriateness, usefulness, and predictability of these tests, either singularly or as part of a battery to replace rabbit eye irritancy testing.

In order to develop the monograph, authors with different expertise contributed sections of the text. These sections were reviewed and redrafted collectively with the anticipation that we represented a spectrum of potential users of the methodologies so that our different perspectives of the problem would be developed within each section. After an extensive literature search, those that had contributed the literature were approached by letter to solicit additional work in progress. The published and unpublished materials were analyzed and critiqued and the draft of the manuscript provided to each of those contacted so that they would be able to comment on the accuracy of the reporting. This should not imply to the reader that a consensus or agreement on the interpretive material developed. The interpretations and criticisms are those of the authors. At the conclusion of the meeting, the manuscript was reedited, along with the development of the summary and the recommendations. These immediately follow.

The book was conceived as a way to examine a series of methods, and to propose an approach for the acceptance of *in vitro* methods as alternatives to eye irritancy testing. It is the anticipation that this volume will be useful to the research and regulatory communities, the industrial and academic scientist and to the lay public that are interested in this specific area.

SUMMARY

This book summarizes the history, current status, and biological basis for in vitro methodology development and provides a comprehensive summary of those methods in the literature that have been identified by

1

the authors of the original papers as replacements for Draize eye
irritancy testing and/or acute ocular cytotoxicity.  It is believed that
this represents a comprehensive review of methodologies that have been
suggested.  It became clear at the workshop and during the writing of
the monograph that no single method developed to date, nor anticipated
in the near future, will provide a replacement for eye irritancy testing
in intact animals.  However, what also has emerged is that it may be
possible to develop a battery of tests which will be useful within
certain industries or for specific categories of products to be tested.

During the preparation of the monograph, several needs, both for new and
fundamental research became apparent.  Alternative or in vitro methods
in the assessment of eye irritancy are innovations.  Like all
innovations, it will take time for these to be used fully.  The use of
animals in toxicity testing will continue to be a major source of data
in meeting regulatory requirements and establishing potential harmful
effects of chemicals.  However, it also is clear at this time that in
vitro methodology already has begun to be used in assessing potential
cytotoxicity and eye irritancy.

NEEDS

Much work must be done if an appropriate battery or batteries of tests
are to be developed to replace eye irritancy testing in animals.  For
presentation here, they have been identified in two categories -
research and validation - and they are listed separately below.

### Research

1.  There is a need to continue to develop new methods for eye
    irritancy evaluation based on fundamental research.  Within
    the subcategories identified for the replacement of
    methodology, be it cytotoxicity or morphology, there is a need
    for the development of improved methodology.  One of the most
    striking needs are for the development of additional methods
    in the area of recovery and repair of ocular damage.

2.  There is a need for the development of understanding of the
    toxico- and pharmacokinetics of materials in in vitro systems
    and their relationship to the in vivo condition.

3.  There is a need for methods to evaluate the response of the
    eye to painful stimuli.  At the present, there have been
    limited studies or developments in the evaluation of pain
    induced by chemicals in the eye in in vitro tests.  There is a
    need to establish correlations between in vivo and in vitro
    sensitivity thresholds, and between the painfulness and
    cytotoxity of various substances.

4.  There is a need to develop both the scientific basis for
    mixture toxicology and for new methods and approaches to
    handle mixtures, solids and water-insoluble material.  It
    appears that most of the methods to date were developed with
    the understanding that the materials to be tested will be
    water soluble.  There has been little development of methods
    which will allow the assessment of complex mixtures, of
    solids, and of water-insoluble materials.

5.  There is a need for quantitative structure-activity
    approaches.  Although empirical approaches to the development

of structure activity relationships have been initiated, there has been little development of quantitative structure activity relationships based on mechanistic understanding.

## Validation

1.  There is a need to more clearly define specific aspects of validation:

    A.  Although it would be desirable to be able to identify a number of specific test protocols, it became clear during the preparation of the monograph that each industry and/or different types of compounds may require the development of distinct and separate batteries of tests. A test battery could be based on the industry, the endpoints to be measured, and/or the chemical and physical properties of the materials to be tested.

    B.  Having identified that separate batteries are necessary, it then becomes apparent that separate standardized chemicals also will become necessary for the validation of these batteries. An additional need, once the identification of compounds is completed, is the necessity to establish a chemical repository to provide these chemicals to investigators.

2.  There is a need to establish a database for chemicals to be used in validation studies. Once the chemicals are identified for validation studies, a substantial and comprehensive database must be developed which will identify known effects in animal species, in in vitro test systems, and from accidental exposure or designed testing trials in humans.

## RECOMMENDATIONS

Four recommendations developed from the preparation of the monograph and workshop. The first is to hold a series of highly structured and coordinated workshops. The second is in the area of validation. The third is for improvements in current in vivo testing. The last is to identify routes for the education of professionals in the area of in vitro methodologies. These recommendations are detailed below.

1.  Three areas have been identified to continue the development of methodology and its validation. These needs can be addressed through workshops which should: (a) identify specific test battery strategies. It was the hope that this book would provide this as an outcome; however, it has become obvious at this early stage in the development of in vitro methods to replace eye irritancy testing this is not yet scientifically justifiable. Additional questions must be answered before test batteries can be specified. However, it is possible to identify strategies in the development of those test batteries; (b) identify specific chemicals to be used in the validation of the tests; (c) define the scientific basis for mixture toxicology and approaches to handling difficult types of materials. These three workshops could be developed along similar lines to those used in the preparation of this monograph as noted in the Preface. Clearly, for each area separate approaches might be needed and it would be expected that the majority of participants in each of the workshops would be different. For the first workshop, each test battery

should be chosen based on the materials to be tested and their anticipated use.

2.  A validation program as described in Chapter 7 of this volume should be initiated for ocular irritancy testing.   There are four phases to validation which should be carried out in sequence.  The first includes:  definition of test objectives, identification of potential alternative tests to meet the defined objectives, and identification of appropriate test chemicals for primary and secondary testing laboratories. This phase for eye irritancy testing is developed in the workshops.  The second phase, microvalidation, involves protocol standardization in the laboratory that developed the test and a preliminary study of 15-20 masked compounds.  Phase three, macrovalidation, involves many laboratories all performing the same assays on 50-100 masked compounds. Macrovalidation establishes the feasibility of technology transfer, the reproducibility of each assay in a test battery and addresses the potential for acceptance of the test battery by the users of the systems.  The final phase will require the optimization or "fine tuning" of a test battery for specific purposes, for the identification of its limitations or exceptions and to optimize the system economically.  With the assays described in this volume, but not limited to them, it is possible to initiate a validation study at this time.

3.  It was recognized that several activities and programs have been under way to update procedures and practices in rabbit eye irritancy testing.  Structuring and further development of these advances should increase and include, when appropriate, additional standardization of protocols based on current state-of-the-art such as low volume testing.  Further decreases in animal use may be accomplished by study designs that include tier approaches to hazard assessment; and the development of ways to share data and to publish all data including results which show no effects.  Improvements in in vivo testing which provides more accurate data and minimizes animal use are strongly encouraged.

4.  In vitro methodology as identified above is an innovation. For an innovation to become utilized effectively, there must be an educational process for those who will use the methodology.  In vitro methodology is commonplace in the research laboratory.  It is less common in routine toxicity testing laboratories.  There is clearly a need for the development of educational and training programs to encourage the use of in vitro methodology.  There thus is a need for the development of short-term, continuing education, and graduate training  of technical, support staff, students and the scientific and regulatory communities.

# Chapter 2

# Historical Perspective
# on Eye Irritation Testing

Early in the 1930s, an untested eyelash dye containing
p-phenylenediamine ("Lash Lure") was brought onto the market in the
United States.  This product (as well as a number of similar products)
rapidly demonstrated that it could sensitize the external ocular
structures, leading to corneal ulceration with loss of vision and at
least one fatality (McCally et al., 1933).  This occurrence, led to the
revision of the law which became the Food, Drug and Cosmetic Act of
1938.  To meet the provisions of this act, a number of test methods were
proposed.  Latven and Molitor (1939) and Mann and Pullinger (1942) were
among those to first report on the use of rabbits as a test model to
predict eye irritation in humans.  No specific scoring system was
presented to grade or summarize the results in these tests, however, and
the use of animals with pigmented eyes (as opposed to albinos) was
advocated.  Early in 1944, Friedenwald et al. published a method using
albino rabbits in a manner very similar to that of the original (1944)
Draize publication, but still prescribing the description of the
individual animal responses as the means of evaluating and reporting the
results.  Though a scoring method was provided, no overall score was
generated for the test group.  Draize (head of the Dermal and Ocular
Toxicity Branch at the Food and Drug Administration) modified
Friedenwald's procedure and made the significant addition of a summary
scoring system.

Over the 40 years since the publication of the Draize scoring
system, it has become common practice to call all eye irritation tests
performed in rabbits "the Draize eye test."  However, since 1944, ocular
irritation testing in rabbits has significantly changed.  Clearly, there
is no longer a single test design that is used and there are different
objectives that are pursued by different groups using the same test.
This lack of standardization has been recognized for some time and
attempts have been made to address standardization of at least the
methodological aspects of the test (such as how test materials are
applied and scoring performed), if not the design aspects (such as
numbers and sources of test animals).  For the purposes of this volume,
we have replaced the term "Draize test" with eye irritancy testing.

The common core design of the test consists of instilling either 0.1 ml of a liquid or 0.1 g of a powder (or other solid) onto one eye of each of six rabbits.  The material is not washed out, and both eyes of each animal (the non-treated eye acting as a control) are graded according to the Draize scale (Table 1) at 24, 48 and 72 hours after test material instillation.  The resulting scores are summed for each

TABLE 1
(Draize, 1944)

SCALE OF WEIGHTED SCORES FOR GRADING THE SEVERITY OF OCULAR LESIONS

I.   Cornea
    A.   Opacity-Degree of Density (area which is most dense is
         taken for reading)
         Scattered or diffuse area-details of iris clearly visible.. 1
         Easily discernible translucent areas, details of iris
            slightly obscured........................................ 2
         Opalescent areas, no details of iris visible, size of
            pupil barely discernible................................ 3
         Opaque, iris visible....................................... 4
    B.   Area of Cornea Involved
         One-quarter (or less) but not zero......................... 1
         Greater than one-quarter - less than one-half............. 2
         Greater than one-half less than three-quarters............ 3
         Greater than three-quarters up to whole area.............. 4
                 Scoring equals A x B x 5     Total maximum = 80

II.  Iris
    A.   Values
         Folds above normal, congestion, swelling, circumcorneal
            ingestion (any one or all of these or combination of
            any thereof), iris still reacting to light (sluggish
            reaction is possible).................................... 1
         No reaction to light, hemorrhage; gross destruction (any
            one or all of these).................................... 2
                 Scoring equals A x B     Total possible maximum = 10

III. Conjunctivae
    A.   Redness (refers to palpebral conjunctival only)
         Vessels definitely injected above normal.................. 1
         More diffuse, deeper crimson red, individual vessels
            not easily discernible.................................. 2
         Diffuse beefy red.......................................... 3
    B.   Chemosis
         Any swelling above normal (includes nictitating membrane).. 1
         Obvious swelling with partial eversion of the lids........ 2
         Swelling with lids about half-closed...................... 3
         Swelling with lids about half-closed to completely closed.. 4
    C.   Discharge
         Any amount different from normal (does not include small
            amount observed in inner canthus of normal animals)...... 1
         Discharge with moistening of the lids and hair just
            adjacent to the lids.................................... 2
         Discharge with moistening of the lids and considerable
            area around the eye..................................... 3
                 Scoring (A + B + C) x 2   Total maximum = 20

The maximum total score is the sum of all scores obtained for the cornea, iris and conjunctivae.

animal. The major subset of variations involve the use of three additional rabbits which have their eyes irrigated shortly after instillation of test material. There are, however, many variations of these two major design subsets (that is, with and without irrigation groups).

Even though the major objective of the Draize scale was to standardize scoring, it was recognized early that this was not happening - that different people were "reading" the same response differently. To address this, two sets of standards (also called training guides, to provide guidance by comparison) have been published by regulatory agencies through the years. In 1965, the Food and Drug Administration (FDA) published an illustrated guide with color pictures as standards (FDA, 1965). In 1974, the Consumer Product Safety Commission (CPSC) published a second illustrated guide (CPSC, 1974) which provided 20 color photographic slides as standards. The Environmental Protection Agency (EPA, 1979) also supported the development of a guide with color plates/slides which is still available from NTIS (Falahee et al., 1981).

A second source of methodological variability has been in the procedure utilized to instil test materials into the eyes. There is now a consensus that the substance should be dropped into the cul-de-sac formed by gently pulling the lower eyelid away from the eye, then allowing the animal to blink and spread the material across the entire corneal surface. In the past, however, there were other application procedures (such as placing the material directly onto the surface of the cornea).

TABLE 2.  SEVERITY AND PERSISTENCE (NAS, 1977)

---

INCONSEQUENTIAL OR COMPLETE LACK OF IRRITATION - Exposure of the eyes to a material under the specified conditions caused no significant ocular changes. No staining with fluorescein can be observed. Any changes that do occur clear within 24 hours and are no greater than those caused by normal saline under the same conditions.

MODERATE IRRITATION - Exposure of the eye to the material under the specified conditions causes minor, superficial, and transient changes of the cornea, iris, or conjunctivae as determined by external or slit-lamp examination with fluorescein staining. The appearance at the 24-hour or subsequent grading of any of the following changes is sufficient to characterize a response as moderate irritation: opacity of the cornea (other than a slight dulling of the normal luster), hyperemia of the iris, or swelling of the conjunctivae. Any changes that are seen clear within 7 days.

SUBSTANTIAL IRRITATION - Exposure of the eye to the material under the specified conditions causes significant injury to the eye, such as loss of the corneal epithelium, corneal opacity, iritis (other than a slight injection), conjunctivitis, pannus, or bullae. The effects clear within 21 days.

SEVERE IRRITATION OR CORROSION - Exposure of the eye to the material under the specified conditions results in the same types of injury as in the previous category and in significant necrosis or other injuries that adversely affect the visual process. Injuries persist for 21 days or more.

---

There also are variations in the design of the "standard" test. Most laboratories observe animals until at least seven days after instillation and may extend the test to 21 days after instillation if any irritation persists.  These prolonged postexposure observation periods are designed to allow for evaluation of the true severity of damage and for assessing the ability of the ocular damage to be repaired.  The results of these tests are evaluated by a descriptive classification scale (Table 2) such as that described in NAS publication 1138 (NAS, 1977), which is a variation of that reported by Green et al. (1978).  This classification is based on the most severe response observed in a group of six non-irrigated eyes, and data from all observation periods are used for this evaluation.

Different regulatory agencies within the United States have prescribed slightly different procedures for different perceived regulatory needs (Gilman, 1982).  These are looked at in more depth in the next section of this review.  There also have been a number of additional grading schemes, but these will not be reviewed here.

# Chapter 3

# Current *In Vivo* Testing Protocols, Procedures, and Practices

Any discussion of current test protocols (or of any proposed in vitro alternatives) must start with a review of why tests are done. What are the objectives of eye irritation testing and how are these different objectives reflected in not just test design and interpretation, but also in the regulations requiring testing and in the ways that test results are utilized.

There are four major groups of organizations (in terms of their products) which require eye irritation studies to be performed. These can be classified generally as the pharmaceutical, cosmetic and toiletries, consumer product, and industrial chemical groups. There also are minor categories (which we will not consider here) such as military agents.

For the pharmaceutical industry, eye irritation testing is performed when the material is intended to be put into the eye as a means or route of application or for ocular therapy. There are a number of special tests applicable to pharmaceuticals or medical devices which are beyond the scope of this volume, as they are not intended to assess potential acute effects or irritation. In general, however, it is desired that an eye irritation test that is utilized by this group be both sensitive and accurate in predicting the potential to cause irritation in humans. Failing to identify human ocular irritants (lack of sensitivity) is to be avoided, but of equal concern is the occurrence of false positives.

The cosmetics and toiletries industry is similar to the pharmaceutical industry in that the materials of interest are frequently intended for repeated application in the area of the eye. In such uses, contact with the eye is common though not intended or desirable. In this case the objective is a test that is as sensitive (as in the preceding paragraph), even if this results in a low incidence of false positives. Even a moderate irritant would not be desired, but might be acceptable in certain cases (such as deodorants and depilatories) where the potential for eye contact is minimal.

TABLE 3

MATRIX OF TEST OBJECTIVES VS. REQUIRED TEST

| TYPES OF ORGANIZATION (Intended Product Use) | DESIRED SENSITIVITY (Lowest level of irritation that it is essential to detect)[1] | FEATURES | | |
|---|---|---|---|---|
| | | NEED TO EVALUATE RECOVERY AND EFFECTS OF TIMELY IRRIGATION | ACCEPTABLE INCIDENCE OF | |
| | | | FALSE POSITIVES | FALSE NEGATIVE |
| Pharmaceutical | Moderate | None | None | None |
| Cosmetic | Moderate | Recovery-High Irrigation-None | Minimal | None |
| Consumer Product[2] (Personal Use) | Moderate | Recovery-High Irrigation-Low | Minimal | None |
| Consumer Product (Household Use) | Substantial | Medium to High | Low | Low for moderates None for substantials |
| Industrial Chemical | Substantial | High | Low | Low for substantials None for severes |

[1] Categories from Table 2

[2] Current FHSA regulations require that any consumer-used product (other than pharmaceuticals and cosmetics, which are regulated by FDA), must be identified as to their potential to cause irritation as defined earlier in this section.

Consumer products which are not used for personal care (such as soaps, detergents and drain cleaners) are approached from a different perspective. These products are not intended to be used in a manner that either causes them to get into eyes or makes that occurrence likely, but because a very large population uses them and the fact that their modes of use do not include active measures to prevent eye contact (such as goggles or face shields), the desire is to identify severe eye irritants accurately. Agricultural chemicals generally fit in this category, though many of them are covered by specific testing requirements under FIFRA.

Finally, there are industrial chemicals. These are handled by a smaller population (relative to consumer products). Eye contact is never intended, and in fact active measures are taken to prevent it. The use of eye irritation data in these cases is to fulfill labeling requirements for shipping and to provide hazard assessment information for accidental exposures and their treatment. The results of such tests do not directly affect the economic future of a material. It is desired to identify moderate and severe irritants accurately (particularly those with irreversible effects) and to know if rinsing of the eyes after exposure will make the consequences of exposure better or worse. False negatives for mild reversible irritation are acceptable.

The needs of these different groups (that is, their test objectives) are summarized in Table 3. To fulfill these objectives, a number of basic test protocols have been developed and mandated by different regulatory groups. Table 4 gives an overview of these as presented previously in part by Falahee et al. (1982). Historically, the philosophy underlying these test designs made maximization of the biological response equivalent with having the most sensitive test. As this review of objectives has shown, the greatest sensitivity (especially at the expense of false positive findings, which is an unavoidable consequence) is not what is universally desired. As shall be seen later, maximizing the response in rabbits does not guarantee sensitive prediction of the results in humans.

Methodological variations that are commonly used to improve the sensitivity and accuracy of describing damage in these tests are inspection of the eyes with a slit lamp and instillation of the eyes with a vital dye (or, most commonly, fluorescein) as an indicator of increase in permeability of the corneal barrier. These techniques and an alternative scoring system, which is more comprehensive than the Draize scale, are reviewed well by Ballantyne and Swanston (1977) and Chan and Hayes (1985).

## TABLE 4

### REGULATORY OCULAR IRRITATION TEST METHODS

| REFERENCE | Draize et al., 1944 | FHSA*, 1964 | NAS*, 1977 | OECD*, 1981 | IRLG*, 1981 | CFR* 16, 1981 (CPSC*) | TOSCA* 1982 | FIFRA*, 1982 (Office Pesticide Assessment) |
|---|---|---|---|---|---|---|---|---|
| Test Species | Albino rabbit | Same | Same[a] | Same | Same | Same | Same | Same |
| Age/weight | NS[b] | NS | Sexually mature/ less than 2 yrs. old | NS | Young adult/2.0 | NS | NS | NS |
| Sex | NS | NS | Either | NS | Either | NS | NS | NS |
| Number Animals/ Group | 9 | 6-18 | 4 (minimum) | 3 (minimum) | 3 preliminary test); 6 | 6-18 | 6 | 6 |
| Test Agent; Volume and Method of Instillation | 0.1 ml on the eye | | | | | | | |
| Liquids | | Same as Draize | Liquids and solid; two or more different doses within the probable range of human exposure | Same as Draize | Same as Draize | Same as Draize | Same as FHSA | Same as FHSA |
| Solids | NS | 100 mg or 0.1 mL equivalent when this volume weighs less than 100 mg; direct instillation into conjunctival sac | Manner of application should reflect probable route of acciden- tal exposure | Same as FHSA | Same as FHSA | Same as FHSA | Same as FHSA | Same as FHSA |

| | | | | | | | |
|---|---|---|---|---|---|---|---|
| Aerosols[e] | NS | NS | Short burst at distance approximating self-induced eye exposure | 1 sec burst sprayed at 10 cm | 1 sec burst sprayed at approx. 4 inches | NS | As OECD | As OECD |
| Irrigation Schedule | At 2 sec (3 animals) and at 4 sec (3 animals following instillation of test agent (3 animals remain non-irrigated) | Eyes may be washed after 24-hr reading | May be conducted with separate experimental groups | Same as FHSA; in addition, for substances found to be irritating; wash at 4 sec (3 animals) and at 30 sec (3 animals) | Same as FHSA | Same as FHSA | As FHSA | As FHSA |
| Irrigation Treatment | 20 mL tap water (body temp.) | Sodium chloride solution (U.S.P. or equivalent) | NS | Wash with water for 5 min using volume and velocity of flow which will not cause injury | Tap water or sodium chloride solution (U.S.P. or equivalent) | Same as FHSA | NS | NS |
| Examination Times (post-instillation) | 24 hr / 48 hr / 72 hr / 4 days / 7 days | 24 hr / 48 hr / 72 hr | 1 day / 3 days / 7 days / 14 days / 21 days | 1 hr / 24 hr / 48 hr / 72 hr | 24 hr[f] / 48 hr / 72 hr | 24 hr / 48 hr / 72 hr | As OECD | As OECD |

TABLE 4 (continued)

REGULATORY OCULAR IRRITATION TEST METHODS

| REFERENCE | FHSA*, 1964 | NAS*, 1977 | OECD*, 1981 | IRLG*, 1981 | CFR 16*, 1981 (CPSC*) | TOSCA* 1982 | FIFRA*, 1982 (Office Pesticide Assessment) |
|---|---|---|---|---|---|---|---|
|  | Draize et al., 1944 |  |  |  |  |  |  |
| Use of Fluorescein | May be applied after the 24-hr reading (optional) | May be used | Same as FHSA | Same as FHSA | Same as FHSA | as FHSA | as FHSA |
| Use of Anesthetics | NS | NS | May be used | May be used | NS | May be used | May be used |
| Scoring and Evaluation | Modified Draize et al., 1944, or a slit lamp scoring system | CPSC, 1976 | CPSC, 1976 | CPSC, 1976 | CPSC, 1976 | (CPSC, 1976) | (CPSC, 1976) |

* FHSA = Federal Hazardous Substance Act; NAS = National Academy of Sciences; OECD = Organization for Economic Cooperation and Development; IRLG = Interagency Regulatory Liaison Group; CFR = Code of Federal Regulations; CPSC = Consumer Product Safety Commission

a Tests should be conducted on monkeys when confirmatory data are required.

b Not specified.

c If the substance produces corrosion, severe irritation or no irritation in a preliminary test with 3 animals, no further testing is necessary. If equivocal responses occur, testing on a least 3 additional animals should be performed.

d Suggested doses are 0.1 and 0.05 mL for liquids.

e Currently no testing guidelines exist for gases or vapors.

f Eyes may also be examined at 1 hr, 7, 14, and 21 days (at the option of the investigator).

In order to develop an approximation of how many rabbit eye irritation tests are performed in the U.S. and how many rabbits are used in the effort, a survey was designed and conducted specifically for this review. One hundred and ninety laboratories were identified as performing such tests in the U.S. and upon examination were classified into three categories which each included approximately a third of total. These categories (called sectors) were contract research labs (58 facilities), pharmaceutical and cosmetic company labs (72 facilities), and chemical company labs (60 facilities, which include the labs of consumer product companies).

A random sample of 10 facilities was then drawn by lot from each of the three sectors. These 30 organizations (representing, it should be noted, 16% of the total population) were then asked to provide information as to how many rabbit eye irritation tests they had performed in the last year, how many rabbits they had used in doing these tests, and what design modifications they might be employing. Specifically excluded were eye tests that were not intended to evaluate irritation. The results of this survey are presented in Table 5.

It should be noted that the "tests" performed annually in Table 5 include a variety of approaches, ranging from two rabbit screens by many of the chemical company labs to a few 48 animal tests (for ophthalmologic agents) by pharmaceutical concerns. Two and three animal tests are screens meant to detect severe irritants (or corrosives) only. This is why they are primarily used by the industrial chemical sector. Reducing the number of animals is not suitable for a test designed to do more than identify extreme and intermediate agents accurately, as this would impair the predictive power of such tests due to the high degree of variability between animals (Bayard and Hehir, 1976).

This estimate of the total number of rabbits used in eye irritation testing is approximately one quarter of the Office of Technology Assessment's estimate of the total number of rabbits used in all biomedical testing. The OTA estimate also includes animals used for dermal irritation and toxicity testing, teratogenicity, reproductive pyrogenicity and pregnancy testing and teaching.

Current in vivo rabbit eye irritation tests also have the perceived advantages of being relatively inexpensive and of requiring minimal time from highly trained personnel. Performing large numbers of tests also leads to a substantial economy of mass effect, with significant reductions in the costs of doing tests. Depending on exactly how the tests are performed and on the local cost of the labor involved, a single material can be evaluated (including compliance with Good Laboratory Practices and the issuing of a final report, which generally account for at least 25% of the effort involved) for a cost of from $400 to $1,600. The times involved range from 10 to 30 person hours per test, with all but a small portion of this effort coming from the most junior technical staff.

In passing, it also should be pointed out that there is a degree of duplication in the testing that is performed - some materials are evaluated by more than one organization. This arises because eye testing data (indeed, all acute testing data) are not generally published. This lack of publication of acute results is due to two causes. First and foremost, the journals of toxicology do not generally believe that such data is of sufficient value to merit publication. The exception is the "battery" publication which presents a large number of results from such tests at one time usually as support for a point of test interpretation or for changing test designs. The second reason

TABLE 5.  RABBIT EYE TESTS

A.  TESTS PERFORMED (ANNUAL)

| SECTOR | RANGE | MEAN (X) | WEIGHTING FACTOR (W) | MEAN FOR SECTOR (X W) |
|---|---|---|---|---|
| Contract | 10-800 | 258 | (58) | 14,964 |
| Pharmaceutical | 0-344 | 65 | (72) | 4,680 |
| Chemical | 28-155 | 83 | (60) | 4,980 |
| | | ESTIMATED TOTAL (E) | | 24,624 |

B.  ANIMALS USED (ANNUAL)

| SECTOR | RANGE | MEAN (X) | WEIGHTING FACTOR (W) | MEAN FOR SECTOR (X W) |
|---|---|---|---|---|
| Contract | 90-4800 | 1520 | (58) | 88,160 |
| Pharmaceutical | 0-1032 | 234 | (72) | 16,848 |
| Chemical | 216-488 | 296 | (60) | 17,760 |
| | | | TOTAL | 122,768 |

W= No. of laboratory in sector is the weighting factor

NOTES TO TABLE 5

Many of the laboratories surveyed reported using alternative techniques or test designs to reduce animal usage and discomfort.  Some of these, in brief, are presented below.

A.  Though one laboratory reported using 48 rabbits in a single eye irritation test, and a number of labs use a 9-animal design (6 non-washed and 3 washed), fully 1/3 of the laboratories use a screen or a sequential test design which reduces the number of animals per test in many (or even most) cases to 2-4 animals.  One lab used both eyes, taking each as an independent variable and thus cutting in half the number of animals per test.

B.  10% of the labs have gone to a 0.01 ml test volume.  Others currently are evaluating this change.

C.  Five labs use the same animals for concurrent dermal and ocular irritation evaluations.  Only one lab used the same animals for more than one eye irritation test - that lab performed a small number of tests.

D.  One-third of the laboratories perform some form of prescreen before performing an eye irritation study.  Prescreens will be discussed later in this section.

E.  Cost per test range from $400 to $1,600 each, depending on the details of the test performed and upon the nature of the personnel employed in performing tests.

such results are not published is concern for the proprietary nature of the materials tested. This concern has abated in recent years and, in fact, should continue to decline.

The rabbit eye irritation test is designed to provide a range of information. First, what kinds of effects are to be expected and how severe are they? The Draize scale was never intended to provide a score such that the data is continuous and linear. That is, a material with a score of 109 is not distinguishable from one with a score of 106. Rather, the results of scoring any one animal were intended to allow an agent to be classified as causing irritation or not in that animal.

Second, the test provides information as to rate of occurrence (or incidence) of irritation in animals. It is actually this information that is used to classify a material as an irritant or not. Under Federal Hazardous Substances Act (FHSA) regulations, for example, this classification process proceeds as follows (Code of Federal Regulations, 1981):

> Interpretation of data is made from six test eyes which are not irrigated with water. Only data from the 24, 48, and 72 hour observations are used for this evaluation. An animal shall be considered as exhibiting a positive reaction if the test substance produces at any of the readings ulceration of the cornea (other than a fine stippling) [grade 1], or opacity of the cornea (other than a slight dulling of the normal luster) [grade 1] or inflammation of the iris (other than a slight deepening of the rugae or a slight circumcorneal injection of the blood vessels) [grade 1], or if such substance produces in the conjunctivae (excluding the cornea and iris) an obvious swelling with partial eversion of the lids [grade 2] or a diffuse crimson-red color with individual vessels not easily discernible [grade 2].

> The test shall be considered positive if four or more of the animals in the test group exhibit a positive reaction. If only one animal exhibits a positive reaction, the test shall be regarded as negative. If two or three animals exhibit a positive reaction, the test is repeated using a different group of six animals. The second test shall be considered positive if three or more of the animals exhibit a positive reaction. If only one of two animals in the second test exhibit a positive reaction, the test shall be repeated with a different group of six animals. Should a third test be needed, the substance will be regarded as an irritant if any animal exhibits a positive response.

Third, what is the time course of response and are any/all adverse effects reversible? Earlier, the criteria for severity and reversibility were presented. Note that if a test is performed so that results (assuming there is irritation) are followed only for 72 hours according to the FHSA guidelines, the only classification of a material that is possible is either irritant or nonirritant.

If one desires to more fully characterize and classify a material in this test system (such as a severe irritant), then one must either continue observations until the responses disappear or to 21 days (at which time most lesions can be determined to be either reversible or non-reversible). In certain cases (if the responses are extreme and test animals are in continued discomfort), a judgment can be made that effects will persist to 21 days.

TABLE 6.  RATIONALE FOR USING RABBIT EYE IRRITANCY TESTS

---

1.  Provide whole animal and organ in vivo evaluation.

    The rabbit test assesses the inflammatory response of a complex
    organ composed of different tissues made up of numerous cell types.
    And when a tissue of an organ becomes inflamed, the whole animal
    responds.

2.  Either neat chemicals or whole products (complex mixtures) can be
    tested.

3.  Either concentrated or diluted products can be tested.

4.  Yield data on the recovery and healing processes.

    A critical factor for a manufacturer to know in order to defend
    against liability suits.

5.  Required screening test of the Federal Hazardous Substances Act.
    (unless data are already available), Toxic Substances Control Act
    and Federal Insecticides, Fungicides and Rodenticides Act (FIFRA).

6.  Quantitative and qualitative test with the Draize Ocular Scoring
    Scale.

7.  Amenable to modifications (irrigation, low volume, anesthetics),
    which will be discussed later.

8.  Extensive data base and cross-reference capability.

9.  The ease of handling of the rabbit.

10. The eye of the albino rabbit presents a large surface of exposed
    globe for observation, and the lack of pigmentation in the iris
    makes it easier to interpret iritis.

11. Test is conservative, providing for maximum protection by erring on
    the side of overprediction of irritancy in man.  With vision being
    a most important sense, a great degree of protection is essential.

---

TABLE 7.  RATIONALE FOR SEEKING ALTERNATIVES TO RABBIT EYE
IRRITANCY TESTS

1.  To reduce or eliminate whole animal and organ in vivo evaluation.

2.  If strict Draize Scale is used, assesses only three eye structures
    (conjunctiva, cornea, iris).

    The Draize Eye Irritancy Test tells us nothing about cataracts,
    pain, discomfort, or clouding of the lens, for example.

3.  Assesses only immediate damage and inflammation produced by
    irritants (not sensitizers, photoirritants, photoallergens).  Note,
    however, that the test was intended to evaluate only acute
    irritation.  The in vivo test also does not evaluate any pain or
    discomfort.

4.  Technician training and monitoring critical (particularly due to
    qualitative nature of evaluation).

    (As it also will be with some in vitro test methods.)

5.  If the objective is either the total exclusion of irritants or the
    identification of severe irritants, rabbit eye tests do not
    perfectly predict results in humans.  Some (such as Reinhardt and
    Schlatter, 1985) have claimed that these tests are too sensitive
    for such uses.  The issue of relative sensitivity will be examined
    later in this section.

6.  There are structural and biochemical differences between rabbit and
    human eyes, which make extrapolation from one to another difficult.

7.  Lack of standardization.

8.  Variable correlation with human results.

9.  Large biological variability.

10. Large, diverse and fragmented data bases which are not readily
    comparable.

Fourth, for many uses, one may wish to know if there is a sensory warning response if a chemical is splashed into the eye. For some materials, such as dimethyl sulfoxide, methyl bromide and bis (2-chloroethyl) sulfate, no stinging or discomfort is caused - just damage to the eye later (Ballantyne and Swanston, 1977).

Finally, will washing or irrigation of the eye (the most common first aid procedure after an accidental exposure) alleviate the effects or make them worse?

What then are the advantages and disadvantages of the current rabbit eye tests in providing this information? The rationale for such tests and for seeking alternatives are presented in Tables 6 and 7 which are modified from those originally proposed by Jackson (1983).

# Chapter 4

# Adequacy of Current
# *In Vivo* Methods

To assess the adequacy of the currently employed eye irritation tests to fulfill the objectives behind their use, we must evaluate them in terms of (1) their accuracy (how well do they predict the hazard to humans), (2) can comparable results be obtained by different technicians and laboratories, and (3) reproducibility and precision within any single laboratory (how well a single lab can repeat tests and accurately evaluate standard or "control" materials). We also should consider what methods and designs have been developed and are being employed as modifications to rabbit eye irritation tests to improve their performance against these criteria.

Assessing the accuracy of rabbit eye irritation tests - or indeed, of any predictive test of eye irritation - requires that the results of such tests can be compared to what happens in man. Unfortunately the human data base available in the literature or resulting from controlled tests is not large. The concerns, however, have been present almost as long as the tests have been performed (Mclaughlin, 1946).

There are substantial differences between the eyes of humans, rabbits and other species. Beckley (1965) presented the following comparison of corneal thickness and area (as a percentage of the total area of the globe) of 4 species, as shown in Table 8.

TABLE 8.   CORNEAL THICKNESS AND AREA

| SPECIES | THICKNESS (mm) | AREA (%) |
|---------|----------------|----------|
| Man     | 0.52-0.54      | 7        |
| Rabbit  | 0.4            | 25       |
| Mouse   | 0.1            | 50       |
| Rat     | about 0.15     | 50       |

Calabrese (1984) presents a comprehensive review of the anatomical and biochemical differences between the ocular systems of humans and rabbits. Other significant differences between rabbit and human corneas have been pointed out by Maurice (1985). First, the rabbit epithelial layer is about 10 times more permeable to hydrophilic solutes than the human, and, second, the threshold to pain of the rabbit eye is much higher than the human, so that irritating substances are likely to be washed away by tears. Both differences will tend to make the rabbit more sensitive.

Many anionic formulations, for example, are severe rabbit eye irritants, but are nonirritants in humans. For other anionics, however, there is moderate human ocular irritation (such as with sodium dodecyl sulfate). However, the relative sensitivities vary from class to class of chemical. Alexander (1965) and Calabrese (1984) both have provided reviews of materials for which rabbits are more sensitive than man. MacDonald et al. (1983) published a review of materials that were both more or less irritant in rabbits than in humans.

In the experience of one of the authors (SCG), reviewing more than 1,000 materials, the prediction of irritancy in humans (as evaluated in medical and poison control center incidence reports) by rabbit eye tests (performed internally) is correct about 85% of the time. Approximately 10% of the time the rabbit test tends to overpredict irritancy, while it underpredicts it less than 5% of the time.

Swanston (1985) also has published a comparative review of 7 different species, including humans. It should be noted that rabbit eye tests do not detect ocular toxicities associated with some ocular anesthetics and eye drops (Andermann and Erhardt, 1983).

The second concern is its reproducibility between laboratories. Weil and Scala (1971) published the most frequently cited study of intra-laboratory reproducibility of eye and skin irritation tests. Twenty-five labs evaluated a battery of 12 materials by a common protocol. The results did show variability between laboratories with a number of labs reporting consistently either more or less severe results than the other labs. A second comparative study, reported on by Marzulli and Ruggles (1973), had 10 laboratories test 7 liquid materials 2 at a time along with a control material. The materials were selected to be intermediate range eye irritants (5 materials) or nonirritants (2 materials). The labs utilized a common set of evaluation criteria, and were found to be quite consistent in properly classifying materials as irritants or nonirritants - a somewhat less stringent comparison of reproducibility than that employed by Weil and Scala (1971). The causes and cures for such variability from lab to lab are multiple, but we already have mentioned differences in methodologies and evaluator training (to name just 2 major sources).

Since the Weil and Scala report, a number of authors like Marzulli and Ruggles (1973) have published comparative studies which have shown a greater degree of reproducibility, though they have not involved as large or diverse a population of evaluators. Some of these are summarized in Table 9 below.

Behind some of these differences in evaluating the reproducibility of the rabbit eye irritation test is a fundamental disagreement as to what these tests should do (or more precisely, what kind of data they should generate). Many believe that the tests should serve to classify materials (into 2 or more categories, such as nonirritants/mild

TABLE 9. SUMMARY OF COMPARATIVE RABBIT EYE STUDIES

| | STUDY | RESULTS | REFERENCE |
|---|---|---|---|
| 1. | 3 materials by 3 readers under 2 separate conditions | 90% reproducibility of irritant/nonirritant classification | Bayard & Hehir (1976) |
| 2. | 7 materials evaluated in duplicate | Tests results reproducible | Williams et al. (1982) |
| 3. | 56 materials evaluated in 3 separate protocols | Each protocol reproducible - variations between tests by different protocols | Guillot et al. (1982) |
| 4. | 29 materials (detergents) evaluated in 2 rabbits, 1 monkey and 1 human test | Results for all non-human models were more severe than man, but low volume rabbit test data were ranked comparable to human data | Freeberg et al. (1984) |

irritants/moderate irritants ...), while others believe it to be critical that a test effectively rank materials.

Several authors have made the point that nonirritants and strong irritants are reproducibly predicted the best. For other materials, several authors have made the point that the use of concurrent reference materials (Gloxhuber, 1985) or twice annual refresher training of readers vs. a set of standards (MacDonald, et al., 1983) improves reproducibility of results and gives a set of standard results against which we can evaluate a drift in test or reading practices.

Finally, the modifications which have been proposed and adapted for the performance of rabbit eye irritation tests themselves should be reviewed. These modifications have been directed at the twin objectives of making the tests more accurate in predicting human responses and at reducing both the use of animals and the degree of discomfort or suffering experienced by those that are used. Some of these modifications already have been discussed (Table 5 and its footnotes).

1.  Alternative Species: Dogs, monkeys and mice (Swanston, 1985) have all been suggested as alternatives to rabbits that would be more representative of humans. Each of these, however, also has shown differences in responses compared to those seen in humans, and pose additional problems in terms of cost, handling, lack of database, etc.

2.  Use of Anesthetics: Over the years, a number of authors have proposed that topical anesthetics be administered to the eyes of rabbits prior to their use in the test. Both OECD and IRLG regulations allow such usage and the CPSC advocates their use. Numerous published (such as Falahee et al., 1982) and unpublished studies have shown that such use of anesthetics can interfere with test results (usually by increasing the severity of eye irritation findings). However, the available literature remains mixed as to

the scientific validity and/or advantages of using anesthetics in
these tests.

Maurice (1955) suggests that anesthesia is an advantage in that it
avoids the stimulation of tear flow by irritants, which is one
cause of variability in the tests.

3.  Decreased Volume of Test Material:  An alternative which has been
    proposed (and which our survey showed has been adopted by a number
    of laboratories) is using a reduced volume/weight of test
    materials.

    In 1980, Griffith et al. reported on a study in which they
    evaluated 21 different chemicals at volumes of 0.1 0.03, 0.01 and
    0.003 ml.  These 21 chemicals were materials on which there was
    already human data.  The volume reduction was found to not change
    the rank order of responses, and it was found that 0.01 ml
    (10 microliters) gave results which best mirrored those seen in
    man.  In 1982, Williams et al. reported a comparison of 7 materials
    evaluated at 0.1 and 0.01 ml and found that the rank of results was
    not changed with the volume reduction while the responses were
    moderated.

    In 1984, Freeberg et al. published a study of 29 detergents (for
    which there was human data), each evaluated at both 0.1 and 0.01 ml
    test volumes in rabbits.  The results of the 0.01 ml tests were
    reported to be more reflective of results in man.

    In 1985, Walker reported on an evaluation of the low volume
    (0.01 ml) test which assessed its results for correlation with
    those in humans based on the number of days until clearing of
    injury and reported that 0.01 ml gave a better correlation than did
    0.1 ml.

    There are only 2 objections to the low volume test.  These are that
    we would lose a screen for exquisitely toxic materials (single
    drops of which in the eye will kill an animal, such as was reported
    for an organophosphonium salt by Dunn et al. in 1982) and that
    there may be some classes of chemicals for which low volume tests
    may give less representative results.

    The American Society of Testing and Materials (ASTM) has published
    the low volume method (Method E 1055-85) as a consensus standard
    procedure.  It seems clear that this approach should be seriously
    considered by those performing in vivo eye irritation tests.

4.  Use of Prescreens:  This modification also may be considered a tier
    approach.  Its objective is to avoid testing severely irritating or
    corrosive materials in many (or, in some cases, any) rabbits.  This
    approach entails a number of steps which should be considered
    independently.

    First is a screen based on physicochemical properties.  This
    usually means pH, but also should be extended to materials with
    high oxidation or reduction potentials (hexavalent chromium salts,
    for example).

    Though the correlation between low pHs (acids) and eye damage in
    the rabbit is not excellent, all alkalis (pH 11.5 or above) tested
    have been reported to produce opacities and ocular damage (Murphy

et al., 1982). This lack of correlation of eye damage and low pHs is not limited to the rabbit, but rather is an inherent property of the more complex chemical reactivities of acids. Many laboratories now use pH cutoffs for testing of 2.0 or lower and 11.5 or 12.0 and higher. If a material falls outside of these cutoffs (or is so identified due to other physicochemical parameters), then it is either (a) not tested in the rabbit eye and assumed to be corrosive, or (b) evaluated in a secondary screen such as an in vitro cytotoxicity test or primary dermal irritation test (Jackson and Rutty, 1985) or (c) evaluated in a single rabbit before a full scale eye irritation test is performed. It should be kept in mind that the correlation of all the physicochemical screen parameters with acute eye test results is very concentration-dependent, being good at high concentrations and marginal at lower concentrations (where various buffering systems present in the eye are meaningful).

The second commonly used type or level of prescreen is the use of primary dermal irritation (PDI) test results. In this approach, the PDI study is performed before the eye irritation study and if the score from that study (called the primary dermal irritation index (PDII) and ranging from 0 to 8) is above a certain level (usually 5.0 or greater), the same options already outlined for physicochemical parameter can be exercised. There is no universal agreement on the value of this prescreen. Gilman et al. (1983) did not find the PDII a good predictor, but made this judgment based on a relatively small data set and a cutoff PDII of 3.0 or above. In 1984 and 1985, Williams reported that severe PDII scores (5.0 or greater) predicted severe eye irritation responses in 39 of 60 cases. He attributed the false positives to possible over prediction of potential human response by current PDI test procedures. On the other side, Guillot et al. (1982 a and b) reported good prediction of eye irritation based on skin irritation in 56 materials and Gad et al. (1986) reported good prediction of severe eye irritation results based on PDIIs of 72 test materials.

5.  Staggered Study Starts: Another approach, which is a form of screen, calls for starting the eye test in one or two animals, then offsetting the dosing of the additional animals in the test group for four hours a day. During this offset period, if a severe result is seen in the first one or two animals, the remainder of the test may be canceled. This staggered start allows one to both limit testing severe eye irritants and yet have confidence that a moderate irritant would be detected.

An integrated summary, the approach presented in these design modifications, is shown in Figure 1. Figure 2 presents the design for the traditional full-scale eye irritation study.

FIGURE 1

# Tier Approach For Eye Irritation Testing

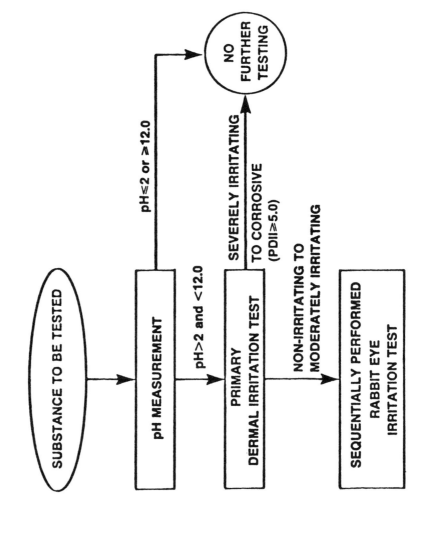

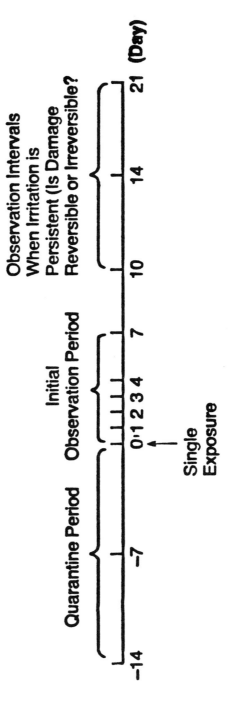

FIGURE 2

Acute Eye Irritation Study

Species: Rabbit
Strain: New Zealand White
Test Group: 9 Animals (6 Nonirrigated; 3 Irrigated)

TABLE 10

MATRIX OF TEST OBJECTIVES AND OPERATIONS

| Objective | Approach | Test Material (Example) | Who is Interested | Goal/Purpose | Regulatory Requirements | Current Status of Reform | Obstacles to Further Reform | Role of Alternatives |
|---|---|---|---|---|---|---|---|---|
| A. Industry: evaluation of irritation/corrosion potential of chemicals not intended to come into contact with the eye and unlikely to do so | Instillation of material into rabbit eye as per Table 4 | Industrial chemical | Manufacturers Users Workers | Hazard awareness Legal (Liability) Labeling | Evaluate and classify potential human injury | Some prescreening being done <br> - pH screens <br> - dermal irritation <br> Low volume tests | Lack of information on in vivo results <br> - no forum for publication <br> - proprietary data <br> "Draize" not standardized <br> Regulations/legal | Allow more intelligent and less extensive use of animals or replace entirely |
| B. Biomedical research: instillation of chemicals in attempt to determine pathophysiology of injury or disease | Instillation of known toxicants into rabbit eye | Known toxicant | Basic scientists | To develop animal models to elucidate disease and formulate therapy for humans and animals | None | Many animal models and in vitro methods in use | Correlations not established between in vivo and in vitro <br> Lack of data | As above |
| C. Determination of toxicity of compounds not intended to come into contact with ocular surface but having an increased risk of doing so | Instillation of material into rabbit eyes in probes or as per Table 4 | Cosmetics Toiletries Consumer product Dermatologics | Manufacturers Marketers Consumers | Formulation and reformulation of product within "acceptable" limits Labeling Legal (Liability) | Label warning – evaluate and classify potential human injury (Market) None premarket | Early experiments Low volume tests | Lack of basic information Correlation with in vivo tests Regulations | Potentially replace animals |
| D. Screening for lack of toxicity of diagnostic or therapeutic compounds | Evaluating for toxicity by instilling in eyes of test species | Topical ophthalmics | Pharmaceutical industry Clinicians Patients | Screening out of toxic formulations and formulation of nontoxic products | Complete information as to potential toxicity required prior to market introduction | Able to screen out in vitro most toxic materials – actual products still require in vivo tests for registration | Lack of basic information Acceptance Capability Expense Regulations | As screens to allow only those products that appear nontoxic to be tested further in animals and then in humans |

## SUMMARY OF REVIEW OF CURRENT TESTING PRACTICES

In summary, the rabbit eye test (as currently employed and practiced) largely fulfills its intended objectives in predicting human ocular irritation. The actual test design and methodologies that have developed over the past 50 years have been employed as the workings of the test system in response to different needs have become better understood. In particular, the last 5 years have seen significant advances in the employment practices of this test (by using various prescreening systems to preclude or severely limit the testing of extremely irritating and corrosive materials) and in actual test conduct (such as changing to a lower test volume to give a result that is both more predictive of human responses in many cases and less discomforting to test animals). These efforts to improve the in vivo test should be encouraged and continued.

Table 10 presents a matrix which compares the different sets of objectives for performing tests with the required features of test operation.

## V.   REFERENCES

Brooks, D. and Maurice, D.  A simple fluorometer for use with a permeability screen.  Alternatives to Animal Testing, Vol. 5., In press.

Maurice, D. and Singh, T. (1986).  A permeability test for acute corneal toxicity.  Tox. Lett. 31:125-130, 1986.

# Chapter 5

# Potential Approaches for the Development of *In Vitro* Alternatives to Eye Irritancy Tests

This section will focus on the development of experimental preparations and methods, and discuss the a priori feasibility of establishing general in vitro models for assessing ocular toxicity and irritancy. Strategies to simulate rabbit eye irritancy tests should include an examination of cytotoxicity, inflammation and repair. While it is not possible to duplicate the complexities of the external milieu, technology has progressed to the point where it is feasible to investigate many of the triggering stimuli underlying these phenomena by using relatively simple cell and tissue preparations in vitro.

It is reasonable to assume that a battery of tests will be required to replace or reduce the use of the rabbit eye irritancy test. The five major areas to consider for the development of protocols include: an examination of cellular morphology; cell metabolism; cellular or tissue physiologic function; the elicitation of inflammatory/immunologic stimuli; and recovery/repair. The selection of specific markers and the development of individual tests for the battery will depend upon the goals of the investigator and the type of tissue chosen for study.

While it is likely that certain endpoints of toxicity will be shared by two or more tests in the battery, it would be advantageous initially to select separate and distinct markers of toxicity for each type of investigation to broaden the understanding of toxic mechanisms. Moreover, individual tests in any battery may not be equivalent or capable of detecting the toxicity of certain types of chemicals, so investigators should include selected tests from several categories for routine screening.

The choice of the cells (or tissue) that should be used for the development of assays is a complicated issue. Cells such as corneal epithelium are relatively difficult to grow in large quantities, and other cells or tissues such as fibroblasts (Shopsis, C., Borenfreund, E., et al., 1984) RBCs, vaginal mucosa (Dubin, N.H., De Blasi, M.C., et al., 1984) and chorioallantoic membrane (Leighton J., Tchao, R., 1985, and Leupke, N.P., 1985) are more readily available. In the latter case,

31

however, measurements are not readily quantifiable and it may be difficult to use the preparation in mechanistic studies.

Decisions regarding the use of particular tissue have to be made by considering the overall goal of the project. Should one consider the measurement of a basal function which is common to all cells, or does one want to evaluate the cytotoxicity that may be seen only in differentiated cells or tissue? Can ocular and nonocular cells be used interchangeably? Is differentiated epithelium the most appropriate tissue to use for in vitro testing? Should one use single or multilayered tissues such as corneal epithelium? And, finally, would it be better to use human or animal cells for initial study?

## MORPHOLOGY

A general approach to the evaluation of in vitro cytotoxicity might include an examination of gross morphology and viability, ultrastructure, adherence and the assessment of the integrity of the plasma membrane.

Gross cellular morphology can be described by phase-contrast microscopy to denote the appearance of cytoplasmic granules, the development of vacuoles, retraction and cell loss, as well as evidence of necrosis. Toxicity might be semi-quantitated by dose-response data from predetermined exposure intervals by measuring the highest tolerated dose (HTD) using a number of different objective criteria (Borenfreund, E. and Borrero, O., 1984, and Takahashi, N., 1982).

The histopathology of cell or tissue cultures also can be evaluated by routine light microscopy using hematoxylin and eosin (H & E), rhodanile blue (Doran, T.I., Vidrich, A., et al., 1980), toluidine blue (Friend, J., Kinoshita, S., et al., 1982), and silver staining (Sun, T.T. and Green, H., 1976), which are three techniques that have been particularly useful for staining corneal epithelium in cell and organ culture. Rhodamine B (Mac Conaill, M.A. and Curr, E., 1964) also can be used to delineate the stratum corneum which can be useful to measure the thickness of the superficial layer.

### Histochemistry

Depletion of intracellular energy stores and accumulation of fatty deposits can be evaluated in tissue by the use of special glycogen and lipid stains such as PAS (Lillie, R.D. and Fullmer, H.M., 1976) and Sudan Black B (Chiffelle, T.L. and Putt, F.A., 1951), or by the fluorescent staining techniques of Kasten et al. (1959) and Popper (1941).

The status of glycolysis and oxidative metabolism in tissue can be evaluated in histologic specimens by dehydrogenase (Baum, J.L., 1963), ATPase (Barritt, C.J., 1981, and Evans, W.H., 1977) and peroxidase (Bell, E., Sher. S., et al., 1983) staining. The disappearance of labile mitochondrial enzymes (Dannenberg, A.M., Jr., Meyer, O.T., et al., 1968, and Lujda, Z., Grossran, R., et al., 1979) and the release of lysosomal enzymes (Namba, M., Dannenberg, A.M., Jr., et al., 1983), which are associated with autolysis, also can be measured by histochemical techniques. Standardization of the latter techniques may provide an ultrasensitive index of tissue injury.

Turnover of phospholipids in experimental preparations can be evaluated by acid Hemastein (Baker, J.R., 1946) and fluorescent techniques (Hawkes, S.P. and Bartholomew, J.C., 1977), which may be of value for assessing damage to plasma membranes. The integrity of the ground substance of the extracellular matrix (ECM) may be assessed by alizarin red or alcain blue (Mowry, R.W., 1975) staining, which may have adjunctive value for determining the degradation of tissue exposed to toxic chemicals that readily penetrate multicellular barriers.

Modifications of fluorescent techniques using acridine orange also have been developed for the visualization of acidic mucopolysaccharides (Saunders, A.M., 1964) and lysosomes (Robbins, E., Marcus, P.I., et al., 1964) which might be useful for detecting the release of nonspecific proteases and its effect on degradation of ECM as a result of cellular injury.

Cellular injury and senescence also can easily be evaluated by identifying lipofuscin (Lillie, R.D., 1956), basophilic (Clark, G., 1981), and acidophilic (Clark, G., 1979) granules in the cytoplasm.

DNA content can be evaluated by a modified Feulgen procedure (Kasten, F.H., 1973) and/or acridine orange (Kasten, F.H., 1981) that differentiates the nucleic acid from RNA. This might be useful for exfoliative studies to evaluate cellular turnover and sloughing. It also might be possible to adapt these techniques for studies by flow cytometry since Grissman et al. (1985) recently have shown that it is feasible to differentiate nuclei acids and protein, using other specific fluorescent dyes.

Most of the histologic techniques that have just been discussed are probably too time consuming to be used for routine testing, but they could be useful in conjunction with vital dye procedures for characterizing the properties of the experimental tissue in vitro, and for making initial estimates of toxicity.

Ultrastructure

Ultrastructural studies by scanning electron microscopy can be used to identify cellular adherence and membrane damage. This technique has been used to evaluate oxidative damage to corneal endothelium in perfused organ cultures (Riley, M.W., 1985), but it has not been widely used for general toxicologic studies.

Transmission electron microscopy, on the other hand, has been used extensively to characterize the early reversible, and the late irreversible changes that take place during cell necrosis. The early reversible changes usually include mild cytoplasmic edema, dilation of the endoplasmic reticulum, minor mitochondrial swelling, disaggregation of polysomes and early perinuclear changes (Wyllie, A.H., 1981, and Trump, B.F., Berezesky, F.K., et al., 1981). The late irreversible changes are typically severe mitochondrial swelling and deformation, gross cytoplasmic swelling accompanied by dissolution of organelles, rupture of the plasma membrane and nuclear lysis (Wyllie, A.H., 1981, and Trump, B.F., Berezesky, F.K., et al., 1981). This might be used appropriately in ocular irritancy studies to evaluate the quality of the apical and basolateral membranes and tight junctions of epithelium; to assess the conditions of the hemidesmosome-basement membrane attachment; and to characterize overall cell polarity. The information that we can get from this type of microscopy warrants its selective use.

Changes in the chemical composition and/or degradation of the ECM also might be localized and evaluated after toxic insult by standard immunofluorescent techniques (Hendrix, M.J.C., Hay, E.D., et al., 1982, and Mayer, B.W., Jr., Hay, E.D., et al., 1981), or by ultrastructural studies of ruthenium red staining after selective digestion of matrix components by glycosidic enzymes (Treslstad, R.L., Hayashi, K., et al., 1974, Hay, E.D., 1978, and Toole, B.P., 1976), and localization of ferritin - and gold-conjugated antibodies which form electron dense complexes with specific constituents of the basement membrane (Horisberger, M. and Rosset, J., 1977). The use of these procedures may be useful in the study of ocular irritancy since the synthesis of hyaluronic acid (HA) appears to be increased in dermal inflammatory reactions and anti-inflammatory steroids decrease the synthesis of HA in cultured fibroblasts (Saarni, H. and Tammi, M., 1978).

## CELLULAR TOXICITY

Cell viability also can be quantitated by the exclusion of vital dyes such as trypan blue or acid violet, or by the uptake of fluorescent dyes such as 4-acetomido-4-isothiocyano-stilbene-2, 2 disulfonic acid (SITS) (Katz, I., 1976) or fluorescein diacetate (Rotman, B. and Papermaster, B.W., 1966). Tissue damage also can be assessed by nitro blue tetrazolium incorporation which is a histologic dye that is normally excluded by the plasma membrane, but stains oxidative enzymes in the cytoplasm of damaged cells (Kaufman, H.E. and Katz, J.I., 1976).

### Adherence

Exfoliative cytology also has been successfully employed in in vitro studies as a qualitative measure of cytotoxicity (Walberg, J., 1983). A quantitative determination of ocular irritancy might be possible by quantifying the number of cells that were shed and/or by normalizing the amount of material that is sloughed to the total amount of DNA or protein in the cell. Another approach that might be used involves the collection of exfoliative cells that are prelabeled with radioisotopes (e.g., $^3$H-thymidine) to measure the rate of cellular turnover by liquid scintillation spectrophotometry. Selective staining of DNA with fluorescent dyes is a third possibility, which would permit an investigator to count the cells by conventional fluorometry or fluorocytometry. The latter techniques have the added advantage in that they are relatively innocuous and could be used repeatedly to evaluate the progression of toxicity over time.

Plating efficiency and growth rate also has been used by some investigators (Hsie, A.W., Schenley, R.L., et al., 1984) as a measure of cytotoxicity after exposure to toxic chemicals.

### Membrane Integrity

The integrity of the plasma membrane is the last parameter we will consider in our discussion of the various facets of general morphology. Lipid peroxidation and permeability changes have been used by most investigators as the 2 classic criteria of damage to the cytoplasmic membrane of cells. Since the role of lipid peroxidation has been associated historically with hepatoxicity (Bridges, J.W., Benford, D.J., et al., 1983), comments will be restricted to the assessment of permeability changes which we consider to be more relevant to irritancy and ocular toxicity.

Permeability changes after exposure to cytolytic or irritative agents can be directly assessed by measuring the leakage of low molecular weight markers such as $^{32}$P(Forbes, I.J., 1963), $^{42}$K (Gale, E.F., 1974, and MacGregor, II., R.D. and Tobias, C.A., 1972), $^{86}$Rb

(Duncan, J.L., 1974, and Hingson, D.J., Massengill, R.K., et al., 1969), $^{42}$K (Madoff, M.A., Cooper, L.Z., et al., 1964); and 2-deoxyglucose (Walum, E., 1982) prelabeled cells, or by the release of endogenous factors and enzymes including ATP (Bergmeyer, H.U., Bernt, F., et al., 1965), NADPH (Henney, C.S., 1973) or LDH (Martz, E., Burakoff, S.J., et al., 1974), which can be used as determination of cell viability.  The leakage of intermediate to high molecular weight markers can be evaluated by prelabeling target cells with precursors that are incorporated into macromolecular synthesis such as $^{14}$C-thymidine (Klein, G. and Peilmann, P., 1963), $^{3}$H-uridine (Thelestam, M. and Mollby, R., 1975 and Thelestam, M. and Mollby, R., 1975), $^{35}$S-methionine (Madoff, M.A., Ortenstein, M.S., et al., 1963), or by $^{51}$Cr (Wigzell, H., 1965) which is generally released bound to cytosolic protein.

The release of $K^+$ is not practical in most systems because of its high spontaneous release, and $^{32}$P, $^{42}$K and $^{86}$Rb are not suitable for routine screening because of their high energy emissions and short half-lives.

Thelestam and Mollby (1976 and 1979) recently have demonstrated that it was possible to prelabel target cells with $^{14}$C-X$_3$aminoisobutyric acid, a metabolically inactive amino acid analogue, and $^{3}$H-uridine to label differentially, low to high molecular weight markers.  By examining the leakage of the amino acid, nucleotides and RNA, the nature of the membrane lesion could be determined.  This is a practical approach that is ideally suited for the rapid screening of primary damage to membrane structure which makes it particularly useful for evaluating the toxicity of surface active agents, such as lipophilic pharmaceutical and industrial chemicals, detergents, and solvents. Cytosolic release easy to quantitate, and a qualitative characterization of membrane damage might be useful for categorizing the mechanism of toxic chemicals.

Moreover, initial chemical injury to the plasma membrane may induce phospholipase A activity which is responsible for the hydrolysis of membrane phospholipids that normally initiate the archidonic acid cascade.  This event is triggered by physical injury or stimulation in many tissues (Bazan, N.G., 1984) including the cornea (Bazan, H.E.P., Birkle, D.L., et al., 1985) and results in the liberation of many prostanoid like substances that are inflammatory and chemotactic to polymorphonuclear leukocytes (PMNs, neutrophils).  An examination of this possibility may be a way to describe primary cellular damage and irritation.  While cytotoxicity, per se, is unquestionably important, its role as a triggering stimulus of inflammatory sequela may have separate significance.

Cellular Metabolism

Aspects of cellular metabolism that might be evaluated by in vitro testing include:  (1) the content of regulatory substances (e.g., Ca$^{2+}$, K$^+$, ATP, cAMP); (2) energy utilization and cell pH; (3) cellular redox status, (4) macromolecular synthesis; and (5) the induction of proteins that may serve as markers of a cellular response to external factors.

The homeostatic control of inorganic ions and adenosine triphosphate (ATP) is one of the most important aspects of cellular metabolism, since they are interdependent and essential for the immediate survival of the cell.  As a consequence, it might be expected that depletion of ATP and perturbation of intracellular ion transport may be one of the features of chemical injury.

Prolonged depletion of ATP may take place as a consequence of impaired synthesis or enhanced destruction.  Inhibition of ATP synthesis may take place by interfering with one or more of the processes or pathways producing reduced cofactors, by depletion of reduced cofactors by futile cycling, or by the inhibition or uncoupling of oxidative phosphorylation.  Interference with ATP levels also may occur by the inhibition of enzymes that are necessary to maintain ATP levels or through the damaging effects of reactive metabolites (Bridges, J.W., Benford, D.J., et al., 1983) which could result in changes in the provision of energy for active transport.

Control of the intracellular concentrations of ions such as $Na^+$, $K^+$, $Ca^{2+}$, $Mg^{2+}$ seem to be essential for cytosolic transport, energy production, macromolecular synthesis, adherence and cell shape, control of cell cycle, and intercellular communication.

The role of calcium influx during the course of cellular injury may be of particular interest since a pronounced elevation of cytosolic $Ca^{2+}$ levels has been associated with a variety of ultrastructural changes and membrane damage, resulting from the release of fatty acids by $Ca^{2+}$-stimulated phospholipases (Holmes, R.P., Mahfouz, M., et al., 1983).  As a consequence, one readily can envision the possibility that the damage induced by the initial chemical injury to the plasma membrane could be extended and amplified by a subsequent rise in intracellular ions which could result in further damage to intracellular structures and the elaboration of inflammatory mediators which could initiate damage in surrounding structures.  Changes in intracellular $Ca^{2+}$, for example, or a modification of the ratios of ATP to adenosine diphoshate (ADP) or reduced to oxidized cofactors, could serve as a sensitive indication of altered membrane permeability and active transport which might be a convenient, reliable marker(s) of the early events leading to tissue destruction and necrosis.  Changes in intracellular ion concentrations can be easily measured by routine atomic absorption spectrometry and perturbations in ATP metabolism can be readily detected by ultraviolet spectrophotometry (Jacobus, W.E., Moreadith, R.W., et al, 1983).

Changes in respiration and glycolysis also can be examined by $O_2$ uptake, and utilization of 1- or 6-$^{14}$[C]-glucose to determine changes in oxidative metabolism, but changes in intracellular pH (Prosad, S.P. and Mukherjee, C., 1983) may be a more practical approach, since intracellular pH generally increases in direct proportion to the level of oxidative phosphorylation.  Neither of these strategies is as convenient as ion measurements, and they probably should be considered as ancillary techniques.

The importance of changes in cellular redox potential in irritancy testing is not clear even though the generation of free-radicals and the redox status of glutathione has been demonstrated to be important in certain types of liver (Bridges, J.W., Benford, D.J., et al., 1983) and corneal toxicity (Whikehart, D.R. and Edelhauser, H.F., 1978, Ng, M.C. and Riley, M.V., 1980, Hull, D.S., Riley, M.V., et al., 1982 and Riley, M.V. and Yates, E.M., 1977).  The analytical methods are easy to use, however, and studies of oxidative damage in cell and organ cultures could be carried out at the investigator's discretion.

Changes in protein and RNA synthesis also can be conveniently examined by radiotracer studies by measuring the incorporation of labeled precursors into macromolecules which may be an advantageous way to evaluate initial toxicity and recovery that has not been fully exploited.

The incubation of target tissue with various $^{14}$C-amino acids or $^{3}$H-uridine after chemical exposure may be an excellent way to evaluate the consequences of cellular injury where damage is unlikely to induce significant changes in the cytoarchitecture of the tissue shortly after contact. Studies by Shopsis, et al. (Shopsis, C. and Sathe, S., 1984, Stark, D.M., Borenfreund, E., et al., 1985, Shopsis, C. and Eng. B., 1985, and Shopsis, C. and Eng, B., 1986) for example, have shown that uptake of $^{3}$H-uridine can be a more sensitive measure of metabolic perturbation than cell proliferation which suggests that this type of protocol may be an excellent strategy for detecting low-grade toxicity before the onset of mitosis and tissue remodeling. Comparable acuity also may be possible using direct measurement of nucleic acid and protein biosynthesis, although this conjecture will have to be confirmed experimentally in parallel studies. The accuracy and resolution of these types of measurements are ideally suited for the rapid screening of ocular toxicants and ranking the potency of irritating chemicals. Because of the rapid collection and analysis of experimental data, it is feasible to use these techniques repeatedly during experimentation to monitor the onset of recovery and the development of protracted toxicity. Since most laboratories currently are equipped to carry out these types of experiments., the reliability of the expanding data base can be assessed quickly by comparing the results of identical projects that have been replicated by a number of different investigators. Significant agreement between laboratories may be an excellent first step toward developing a broad classification schema of toxic chemicals by considering the duration of residual affects. The duration of the toxic response and its impact upon healing is likely to be very important for risk assessment and the proper choice of medical treatment following intentional or accidental exposure.

The measurement of qualitative and quantitative changes in the synthesis of specific proteins may be a more refined strategy for evaluating cytotoxicity and cellular damage which is based upon the premise that cells respond to perturbations in their environment by altering a broad spectrum of biochemical processes. An approach to the evaluation of inducible synthetic pathways could include an examination of cellular repair processes, protective or detoxification mechanisms, and the induction of structural and cell-surface proteins that are inherent to the proliferative process.

Activation of enzymes essential to cellular repair (Schlesinger, M.J., Ashburner, M. and Tissieras, A., 1982, and Dunkel, V.C., 1983) and kinetic detoxification (Frazier, J.M., 1985, and Williams, T., 1959) have been demonstrated to be common characteristics of many cell types that have been subjected to various types of environmental, genomic, and chemical stress. It is tempting to postulate that similar inducible pathways may exist to prevent or retard the deleterious consequences of acute chemical injury on cellular metabolism and membrane transport. The elicitation of this type of feedback might be analogous to the metabolic arrest and the stabilization of membrane function which is a defensive strategy against hypoxia and hypothermia, and a typical metabolic adaptation which can be observed during hibernation (Hochochka, P.W., 1986).

Another avenue for investigation is an examination of the induction of structural and membrane proteins in epithelium which appears to be intimately involved in the migration and proliferation of tissue during the healing process. Studies of this nature using cell or organ cultures could prove to be relevant to the evaluation of acute irritation where it might be difficult to ascertain the extent of injury

or to determine whether the basal cell layer or the ECM has been
damaged.

While a great deal is known about the morphology of epithelial
migration, it has been only in the last several years that an
understanding of some of the biochemical events that occur during the
movement of the epithelial sheet to repair and cover the wounded area
and reattach to the basement membrane.  Epithelial injury generally
seems to result in a retraction of the corneal epithelium away from the
wound which is normally followed by an extension of filopodia and
lamellopodia onto the denuded corneal surface (Haik, B.C. and Zimny,
M.L., 1977, Pfister, R.R., 1975, and Brewitt, H., 1979).  Active cell
migration is typically apparent within 4 hours of wounding and
progresses at a rate of 26-60um/hr until the wound closure is complete
(Kuwabara, T., Perkins, D.G., et al., 1976, and Buck, R.C., 1979).
During reepithelization, small defects are covered by the migration of
adjacent cells which reduces the thickness of the epithelial layer
covering the wound.  Gipson and her colleagues (1980 and 1982) have
shown that enhanced glycoprotein synthesis is exhibited by migrating
epithelium and the synthesis of glycoprotein is essential for complete
wound healing.  Moreover, lectin binding is more intense in migrating
cells which suggests that the cell surface sugars of migrating sheets is
different from normal tissue (Gipson, personal communication).  These
observations imply that there is a change in the cell surface markers
during the transition from stationary to migration which could provide
some excellent metabolic markers of cellular damage and hyperplasia.
This phenomenon may be a general response of epithelium, since
intestinal (Etzler, M.E. and Branstrator, M.L., 1974), buccal
(Dabelsteen, E., et al., 1982) and cutaneous (Brabec, R.K., et al.,
1980) epithelial cells also exhibit similar changes in lectin binding
during differentiation and migration.

Actin filaments and a functioning glycolytic pathway also are
necessary for cell migration (Gipson, I.K. and Anderson, R.A., 1977,
Gipson, I.K., Westcott, M.J., et al., 1982, Gipson, I.D. and Keezer, L.,
1982, and Byers, H.R. and Fujiwara, K., 1982).  Stress fibers have been
observed in vitro and in situ (Byers, H.R. and Fujiwara, K., 1982), and
appear to be important in cell migration (Lazarides, E. and Weber, K.,
1974, and Goldman, R.D., Schloss, J.A., et al., 1976), changes in
cellular shape (Henderson, D. and Weber, K., 1979), and adhesion to the
substrate (Lazarides, E. and Weber, K., 1974, and Wehland, J., Osborn,
M., et al., 1979).  Moreover, disruption of epithelial cell
microfilaments has been implicated as the underlying cause of
persistent, nonhealing epithelial defects that have been observed in
clinical cases resulting from chronic usage of topical anesthetics and
beta-blockers (Burns, R.P., Forster, R.K., et al., 1975, Van Buskirk,
E.M., 1979, Van Buskirk, E.M., 1980, and Nork, T.M., Holly, F.J., et
al., 1984).  Since the maintenance of microfilaments is thought to be
dependent on calmodulin (Burns, R.P., Forster, R.K., et al., 1975), the
kinetics of this important calcium-binding regulatory protein could
provide an excellent marker of acute and chronic toxicity.
Investigators should be cautious about using it in screening tests,
however, since Soong and Citron (1985) have shown that epithelial
migration in the rabbit is not calmodulin-dependent.  In the rabbit,
migrating cells are devoid of stress fibers and cytoplasmic extensions
which indicates that structures are not necessary for motility.
Although the biologic implication of species difference is unknown,
their observations imply that the choice of species (and possibly target
tissue) can be critical when considering the use of a particular
endpoint of toxicity.

On the other hand, microtubule assembly and mitosis do not appear to be necessary for cellular migration in any of the species that have been examined (Gipson, I.K. and Anderson, R.A., 1977, and Gipson, I.K., Westcott, M.J., et al., 1982). Although the precise stimulus that initiates cell migration is unknown, evidence suggests the generation of AMP as a intracellular secondary messenger (Jumblatt, M.M., Fogle, J.A., et al., 1980, and Jumblatt, M.M. and Neufeld, A.H., 1981). Quantitative determinations of cAMP or a change in its metabolism might provide another excellent metabolic marker which can be used in the screening of ocular toxicity.

When the basement membrane is damaged or destroyed during ocular injury, wound closure appears to be followed by synthesis of a new basement membrane by the confluent epithelium (Kenyon, K.R., 1969, and Kenyon, K.R., Fogle, J.A., et al., 1977). In situations where the ocular damage is severe, the elaboration of various collagens and glycoproteins such as fibronectin and laminin, which are normal constituents of the ECM, could be monitored quite easily by conventional radiotracer studies and immunofluorometry. This type strategy might be an excellent way to define the extent of damage and the persistence of any epithelial defect after exposure to ocular irritants. Elaboration of the basement membrane also is closely coupled with the formation of new hemidesmosomes junctions. The time course of these events offers the possibility that the synthesis of specific protein components of the junctional complexes also could be used as ancillary markers of time remodeling. Complete re-epithelization is characterized by a return to its normal multilayered state with a normal distribution of hemidesmosomes that anchor the epithelium to the underlying stroma.

There also is substantial evidence to indicate that the process of corneal regeneration is likely to involve a change in the state of epithelial growth and differentiation which leads to the possibility that the expression of keratins also may be a useful indication of healing and recovery. The expression of keratins, which are the major cytoskeletal proteins of all epithelial cells (Franke, W.W., Appelhaus, B., et al., 1979, Sun, T.T. and Green, H., 1978, and Sun, T.T., Shih, C., et al., 1979), is known to be dependent on its state of differentiation (Fuchs, E. and Green, H., 1980, Sun, T.T. and Green, H., 1977, and Franke, W.W., Schiller, D.L., et al., 1981). Jester et al. (1985) have shown recently that there is a change in the expression of keratins during corneal epithelial healing in rabbits. In that particular study, they found that the expression of two specific keratins (48/56Kd) was associated with cell migration and rapid proliferation. Since other investigators have demonstrated that these same proteins also can be found in cultured skin, corneal and conjunctival epithelial cells (Doran, T.I., Vidrich, A., et al., 1980, Fuchs, E. and Green, H., 1980, and Sun, T.T., and Green, H., 1977), they suggested that the 48/56Kd keratins can be regarded as markers of proliferating keratinocytes. The expression of these keratins persisted in vivo until the epithelial cells reattached to the underlying cornea and reestablished a normal distribution of hemidesmosomal functions with the basement membrane. The latter observation may be important to the evaluation of ocular toxicity, since it implies that the appearance (or absence) of these two proteins could then be used to delineate the point of complete recovery following chemical injury.

In general, studies of intracellular metabolism probably permit a more sensitive assay or measure of the health of the tissue. Some metabolic perturbations may prove to be too sensitive in that some substances may alter to a minimal but measurable extent with metabolism but not significantly affect "normal function or morphology" and, therefore, be of no real consequence in terms of acute toxicity. However, metabolic studies may be crucial in defining chronic toxicity.

CELL AND TISSUE PHYSIOLOGY

Any consideration of physiologic parameters will depend on the tissue in question and its normal function. The cell layer of major importance in irritancy testing is the ocular surface epithelium, i.e., conjunctiva and cornea. To a lesser extent, the conjunctiva substantia propia and corneal stroma and endothelium are of importance; however, a nontoxic substance should not penetrate through the epithelium which normally has a strong barrier function. As a consequence, these comments will be restricted to epithelial preparations.

A number of experimental preparations can be devised to examine ion pump activity, barrier function and the maintenance of electrical potentials of epithelial cells in vitro. The $Na^+$ and $Cl^-$ pump of corneal epithelium in organ culture can be readily evaluated in perfusion chambers maintained under controlled conditions (Klyce, S.D. and Crosson, C.E., 1985). The technology is well established, but the procedure is cumbersome to use for routine screening, and the large number of donor corneas that would be needed would not appreciably reduce the number of animals required. The use of isolated epithelium grown on semipermeable membranes which can be mounted in a modified dual chamber, Boyden chamber, is another approach which has not been tried for routine screening, although this type of preparation is under active development in the laboratory of the authors (JM and DRM). It may be possible to grow and maintain corneal (or conjunctival) epithelium on fixed gelatin membranes (Schwartz, B.D. and McCulley, J.P., 1981), coated chemotactic filters (Taylor, R.F., Price, T.H., et al., 1981) or retracted collagen gels containing viable fibroblasts (Prunerieras, M., Reginier, M., et al., 1983), among other possibilities.

Changes in barrier function also can be examined by measuring the penetration of fluorescent dyes, e.g., fluorescein, or radiolabeled molecular weight markers through the epithelium of mounted whole corneas (D. Maurice, Personal Communication), or in situ by using proptosed eyes of freshly killed mice. Studies of barrier function by measuring penetration of defined molecular-weight markers through epithelial layers maintained on semipermeable supports would be a great advantage, provided the cells develop an effective barrier that approximates the in situ conditions. Measuring the permeability of $^3$H-inulin, $^{14}$C-mannitol and various $^{125}$I labeled proteins of graded molecular weights is an example of one approach that would permit investigators to estimate the volume of the extracellular space and evaluate the relative contribution of paracellular and transcellular invasion as a consequence of the breakdown of the normal epithelial barrier. Epithelial preparations grown on gels containing viable fibroblasts may be particular well-suited for these types of studies, since it is known that fibroblasts release many inflammatory and chemotactic mediators and may influence the integrity and permeability of the epithelium (Bazan, H.E.P., Birkle, D.L., et al., 1985, Grabner, T., Sinzinger, H., et al., 1984, Eliason, J., Deshmukh, A., et al., 1984), may provide a closer simulation of the in vivo condition.

Changes in electrical resistance and the maintenance of the transepithelial potential may be from microelectrode recording from intact corneas or epithelium grown on the various types of semipermeable supports. Measurement of intracellular potentials of corneal epithelium grown on the surface of plastic culture dishes also may be useful, since the cells can be maintained as a differentiated tissue (Franke, W.W., Schiller, D.L., et al., 1981, Chan, K.Y. and Haschke, R.H., 1981, and Chan, K.Y. and Haschke, R.H., 1982).

In essence, the adaptation of confluent layers of differentiated epithelium grown on semipermeable supports would be an ideal preparation for evaluating several distinct physiologic characteristics. Utilization of this type of preparation is likely to be less cumbersome and time-consuming than using isolated corneas. Furthermore, the need for animals would be reduced and the simplicity of the preparation may result in more consistent experimental data.

## INFLAMMATION/IMMUNITY

There are many stimuli and pathways to consider, including specific immunologic factors and manifestations of cytotoxicity which result in the nonspecific release of a variety of inflammatory and chemotactic factors. There is a corresponding activation and release of proteolytic enzymes which affect vascular tone and permeability, promote neovascularization and cellular infiltration, and the degradation of tissue and extracellular matrix. By developing cell and tissue preparations which can be used in predictive in vitro screening, it should be possible to identify and determine the best way to quantitate a few of the representative markers of these phenomena.

Humoral and cellular immunologic responses probably are not relevant to acute toxicity, but they would play a role in the allergic inflammatory response induced by ocular irritants in previously sensitized individuals. Therefore, it might be useful to develop in vitro tests to screen for compounds which have unusual sensitization potential. The development of this type of strategy is beyond the scope of this volume, however, and we will not review this phenomenon here.

The local cytolytic effect of ocular irritants probably is a more relevant concern, since the typical contact of irritating chemicals can result in extensive membrane damage and the activation of the archidonic acid cascade which is initiated by the hydrolysis of membrane phospholipids by phospholysiase $A_2$. This event is triggered by injury or trauma in many tissues (Bazan, N.G., 1970), including the cornea (Bazan, H.E.P., Birkle, D.L., et al., 1985), but the phenomenon has not been studied in relation to ocular toxicity or chemical irritation. Since it is well established that corneal and conjunctival epithelium and fibroblasts are capable of the synthesis and release of cycloxygenase (Bazan, H.E.P., Birkle, D.L., et al, 1985, Leopold, I.H., 1982, Weissman, G., 1980, and Kulkarni, P.S. and Srivivasin, B.D., 1981) and lipoxygenase (Bazan, H.E.P., Birkle, D.L., et al., 1985, Leopold, I.H., 1982, Weissman, G., 1980, and Bazan, E.P., Birkle, D.L., et al., 1985) products which have potent inflammatory and chemotactic properties, the use of these cells in vitro screening may provide an excellent assay system for the detection of ocular irritancy (see Figure 3).

Moreover, the differential metabolism of prostanoids via the cyclooxygenase pathways also may result in a corresponding production of oxygen radicals which could synergistically enhance the inflammatory effects of other prostaglandins (Dubin, N.H., 1985). This suggests that a qualitative characterization of archidonic metabolites may permit investigators to make a more refined distinction between groups of suspected irritants. Prostaglandins and their metabolites can be measured conveniently by standard commercially available RIA procedures and leuckrotrienes and the hydroxymetabolites of archidonic acid can be

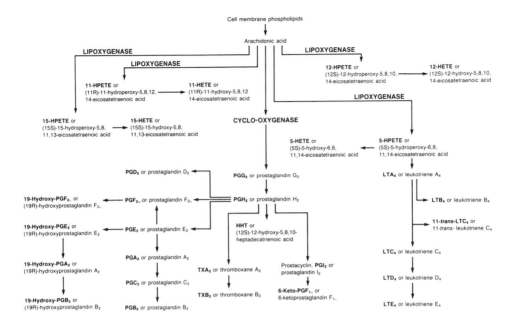

Figure 3

Activation of the archidonic acid cascade showing the synthesis and
metabolism of prostaglandin endoperoxides, thromboxanes, protacyclin and
leukotrienes. The production of endoperoxides of the $PGG_1$ and $PGH_1$
series from the hydrolysis of dihomo-y-linolenic acid are not shown.
(Slightly modified from N.A. Nelson et al., Chemical and Engineering
News 60:30, 1982).

detected and monitored by a number of HPLC techniques (Bazan, H.E.P.,
Birkle, D.L., et al., 1985, Chang, J., Liu, M.C., et al., 1982, Rouzer,
C.A., Scott, W.A., et al., 1982, and Rouzer, C.A., Scott, W.A., et al,
1981).

Furthermore, the recent observations of Bazan, et al. (1985) who
have demonstrated that there are different profiles of archidonic acid
metabolism in the various cellular layers of organ-cultured corneas,
suggests that experimental preparations of epithelium in semipermeable
supports may have several advantages over conventional tissue cultures.
An identified need is the development of epithelium grown on collagen
gels impregnated with viable fibroblasts and/or chemotactic membranes
with or without surface of corneal endothelial cells. The problems that
might be encountered in developing this type of in vitro propagation
should not be too difficult to solve. The results of experiments
utilizing these types of preparations may provide a closer simulation of
in vivo conditions, especially if ocular irritants induce a markedly
different synthetic response in the various tissues.

Another approach is suggested by the fact that inflammation and
cellular infiltration also may be controlled by the release of a variety
of nonprostanoid chemotactic substances by the injured tissue which are
generally known as leukocyte chemotactic factors (LCF) and vascular
endothelial chemotactic factors (VCEF) (Wilkinson, P.C., 1982, Keller,
H.U. and Till, G.O., 1983, Elgebaly, S.A., Nabawi, K., et al., 1985,
Gallin, J.I. and Quie, P.G., 1978, Rowland, F.N., Donovan, M.J., et al,

1983, Klintworth, G.K., 1973, and Klintworth, G.K. and Burger, P.C.,
1983). Moreover, recent studies by Elgebaly, S.A., (Klintworth, G.K.
and Burger, P.C., 1983, Elgebaly, S.A., Forouhar, F., et al., 1984,
Elgebaly, S.A., Gillies, C., et al, 1985, and Fromer, C.H. and
Klintworth, G.K., 1976) have shown that leukocytes are capable of
damaging corneal tissue in animals and in vitro. It is likely that
developing protocols to measure the release of these substances by using
preparations such as a corneal cup, cell cultures, or epithelium grown
on semipermeable supports, could provide another strategy for in vitro
screening. The release of chemotactic factors after exposure to toxic
agents can be detected by bioassay using PMN or macrophage chemotaxis in
Boyden chambers (Stark, D.M., Shopsis, C., et al., 1983 and Shopsis, C.,
Borenfreund, E., et al., 1985), but the chemical characterization of
substances in the future might permit the development of more refined
RIA or ELISA procedures which would be more quantitative and less time
consuming.

Chemotaxis also may be elicited by the degradation of various
components of the ECM. West et al. (1985) recently reported that
degradation products of sodium hyaluronate are angiogenic in a
chorioallantoic membrane assay. It might be possible to study the
formation and release of degradation products with chemotactic
properties by using cells that are grown on the denuded basement
membrane produced by cultured bovine corneal endothelium (Gospodarowicz,
D. and Tauber, J.P., 1980), rabbit epithelium (Sundar-Raj, C.V.,
Freeman, I.L., et al., 1980) or embryonic chick tissue (Sugrue, S. and
Hay, E.D., 1982, and Sugrue, S. and Hay, E.D., 1981), as targets for
irritancy testing. It also is conceivable that cell-free assays could
be developed by using the denuded ECM, per se, for exposure to the
irritant chemicals. Release of degradation products could be measured
conveniently by radiotracer studies by using ECMs that are prelabeled
with incorporated $^3$H-proline or $^3$H-glucosamine by conventional
procedures and subsequent bioassay of their chemotactic properties.

Degradation of the ECM and tissue remodeling also may be regulated
by the activation and release of a variety of exoenzymes at the site of
injury which has implications for a third strategic approach to in vitro
testing.

The fibrolysis that often accompanies tissue injury in the cornea
probably is related to the production and release of plasminogen
activator (PA) (Lantz, E., Dyster-Aas, K., et al., 1978, and Pandolfi,
M. and Lantz, E., 1979) which has been demonstrated in alkali-burned
corneas in vivo and in vitro (Berman, M., Leary, R., et al., 1980, and
Berman, M., Winthrop, S., et al., 1982). Measurement of PA release by
epithelial cultures after exposure to toxic substances has been the
approach taken by Chan (1985), based upon the assumption that the
liberation of the serine protease is critical to the onset of cellular
migration and the initiation of tissue remodeling.

Systemic and localized inflammation of the eye (Berman, M., 1980)
and other tissues (Vaes, G., 1980) also may be provoked and exacerbated
by the liberation of collagenase and nonspecific neutral proteases from
epithelium, fibroblasts and other meschysmal cells within the tissue
which may be modulated by macrophages and ultimately under control of
the immune system. Berman et al. (1983 and 1985) recently demonstrated
that epithelial release of latent collagenase can be activated in
alkali-burned corneas, which suggests that this enzyme may be an
appropriate marker for in vitro screening. The earlier efforts of
Muller and Gross (1978) have indicated that fibroblasts are necessary

for the secretion and release of collagenase by epithelium which implies that cell cultures of epithelium cocultured with fibroblasts, or grown on semipermeable supports could be an ideal experimental preparation for use in these types of assays. The release of collagenase can be measured conveniently by commercially available RIA procedures or assayed by using radiolabeled collagen as a substrate (Muller, B.J. and Gross, J., 1978). Nonspecific protease activity also can be assayed by conventional spectrophotometry using a variety of substrates or quantitated by liquid scintillation counting by measuring the release of specific components of the ECM which have been prelabeled with incorporated radiotracers.

The potential also exists for using an inflammatory effector cell as an in vitro target to predict non-cytotoxic induced inflammation. In such a system, the target cells would be exposed to test substances and the bathing medium would be assayed for a putative released mediator. A test or tests of the propensity of a substance to produce inflammation is of utmost interest to the development of an alternative to rabbit eye irritancy tests. The initial steps in the production of inflammation are not clear (except cytotoxicity); therefore, a by-product must be measured. At this time, it would seem that a direct measure of prostanoid release, assay for chemotactic factors, assay or measurement of exoenzymes, or assay of some other non-specific inflammatory mediator is likely to be fruitful.

### RECOVERY/REPAIR

Generically, these phenomena can be determined in one of two ways: (1) either observe the experimental tissue in question after it has been exposed to the chemical irritants for recovery, by monitoring the same morphologic or biochemical marker that was used to establish "toxicity"; or (2) by wounding the tissue and observing its repair in the presence of the substance in question.

The latter probably is simply another measure of cytotoxicity with some physiologic considerations. This may be a very good, if not the best system, to enable investigators to evaluate this type of interaction. This is similar to the type of strategy that currently is being developed by Jumblatt and Neufeld (1985 and 1986) who are damaging epithelial cells by a standardized cryogenic wound in order to evaluate the effect of various chemicals on wound closure.

The former approach could be applied to almost any of the "assays" listed in the chapter and it may be important to incorporate an evaluation of recovery as an adjunctive test with any of the adopted protocols.

# Chapter 6

# Critical Evaluation
# of Alternative Tests

The fundamental purpose of this report is to evaluate the status of currently proposed in vitro test systems that are intended to replace the rabbit eye irritancy test in predicting human risk of ocular irritation and inflammation resulting from exposure to chemical agents. The basic question simply reduces to asking whether or not the available knowledge and technology base are adequate for this purpose. Before establishing the criteria for such an evaluation it may be beneficial to examine the operational characteristics of an "ideal" test. The purpose of such an exercise is to identify clearly the important mechanical qualities of a test system which should be taken into consideration in any critical evaluation. While considering each of these "ideal" test characteristics the reader should evaluate how well the Draize eye test would measure up to these criteria.

Any useful test system must be sufficiently sensitive that the incidence of false negatives is low. Clearly a high incidence of false negatives is intolerable. In such a situation, large numbers of irritating or corrosive chemical agents would be carried through extensive additional testing only to find that they possess undesirable toxicological properties after the expenditure of significant time and money. On the other hand, a test system which is overly sensitive will give rise to a high incidence of false positives which will have the deleterious consequence of rejecting potentially beneficial chemicals. The "ideal" test will fall somewhere between these two extremes and thus provide adequate protection without unnecessarily stifling development.

The "ideal" test should have an endpoint measurement which provides continuously variable parametric data such that dose-response relationships can be obtained. Furthermore, any criterion of effect, i.e. ED50, must be sufficiently accurate in the sense that it can be used to reliably resolve the relative toxicity of two test chemicals which produce similar responses. In general, it is not sufficient to classify test chemicals into generic toxicity categories, such as "intermediate" toxicity, since a test chemical which falls in a given category, yet is borderline to the next more severe toxicity category, should be treated with more concern than a second test chemical which falls at the less toxic extreme of the same category. Therefore, it is useful for a test system to be able to rank test chemicals accurately within any general toxicity category.

The endpoint measurement of the "ideal" test system must be objective. This is important so that a given test chemical will give similar results when tested using the standard test protocol in different laboratories. If it is not possible to obtain reproducible results in a given laboratory over time or between various laboratories, then the historical database against which new test chemicals are evaluated will be time/laboratory dependent. Along these lines, it is important for the test protocol to incorporate internal standards to serve as quality controls. Thus, test data could be represented utilizing a reference scale based on the response to the internal controls. Such normalization, if properly documented, could reduce inter-test variability.

The test results for a given chemical should be reproducible both intrinsically (within the same laboratory over time) and extrinsically (between laboratories). If this condition is not satisfied, then there will be significant limitations on the application of the test system since it could potentially produce conflicting results. From a regulatory point of view this possibility would be highly undesirable.

Alternatives to the in vivo eye tests basically should be designed to evaluate the acute toxic response of the occular system following a single exposure to the test chemical. Although there are certain variations of the Draize eye test utilized to evaluate repeated exposures to a test agent, this is not the basis of the original test. However, for agents which may enter the conjunctival sac repeatedly, such as facial cosmetics, it would be desirable if the test protocol could be modified to accommodate such an exposure regime. This would certainly be a useful property of a test protocol, but not an essential feature.

From a practical point of view, there are several additional features of the "ideal" test which should be satisfied. The test should be rapid so that the turnaround time for a given test chemical is reasonable. Obviously the speed of the test and the ability to conduct tests on several chemicals simultaneously will determine the overall productivity. The test should be inexpensive so that it is economically competitive with current testing practices. And finally, the technology should be easily transferred from one laboratory to another without excessive capital investment for test implementation. It should be kept in mind that although some of these practical considerations may appear to present formidable limitations for a given test system at the present time, the possibility of future developments in testing technology could overcome these obstacles.

This brief discussion of the characteristics of the "ideal" test system provides a framework for evaluation of alternative test systems in general. No test system is likely to be "ideal." Therefore, it will be necessary to weigh the strengths and weaknesses of each proposed test system in order to reach a conclusion on how "good" a particular test is. The next section will present the basis for the specific test evaluations.

CRITERIA FOR TEST EVALUATION

Many test systems described in the scientific literature (Table 11) have been proposed as alternatives to eye irritancy testing. In order to compare these potential alternative tests it is necessary to establish a set of yardsticks which can be used to evaluate each test system. This section describes the criteria which were developed for this purpose.

The actual evaluation of each test system is divided into 3 categories: (I) logistics, (II) scientific and (III) economic.

(I) Logistics: For a test system to be of practical use it is essential that it meet criteria with respect to: its ability to be standardized; whether it is transferable between laboratories; and whether components of the system are available commercially. Although at first glance these three aspects appear to be independent they are in fact strongly interdependent. The greater the ability to standardize a test protocol the more easily it can be transferred between laboratories. If components of the test system are available commercially, it will be more easily standardized. Thus, we find that there is a strong relationship between commercial availability of components of the test system and whether it meets the logistics criteria.

From the logistical point of view, most test systems can be divided into two components: the biological component and the non-biological component. The biological component is the cell culture, tissue or organ which is used to evaluate the toxicity of the chemical agent. The non-biological component consists of everything else and can be subdivided into those elements which support the biological component and those elements which are involved in the endpoint evaluation. It should be noted that the non-biological components of a test system may include materials derived from biological systems, such as fetal calf serum or antibodies. In the analysis which follows, each of these components is evaluated as to its availability and standardization.

(II) Scientific: This portion of the evaluation looks at the scientific merit of the test system. The first question to be addressed is the nature of the test; i.e., does the endpoint measured evaluate a critical step in the inflammatory/irritation response - mechanistic based test; or does it measure a parameter which merely correlates with the response - correlation based test. This is an important point in terms of acceptance of the test by regulatory agencies since mechanistic tests will be more readily interpretable. Secondly, the endpoint of the test will be evaluated as to whether it is subjective or objective. If it is subjective then the grading scale will be evaluated. The second step in the scientific evaluation is to determine the performance of the test as measured by its correlation with the results of the in vivo eye test in either animals or man. This allows a comparison to be made with a relatively large database in the case of animal data and, where the data are available, the results for a given test will be correlated with the human experience. In general, these data are compared on the basis of rank correlations. No attempt will be made to correlate these data on a quantitative basis.

(III) Economics:  This section deals with factors which determine the cost of the test system. The major components of the analysis include the operational cost of the test per full evaluation of a specific test chemical, the time it takes to carry a test chemical

Table 11
LIST OF TEST PROTOCOLS

A.  Morphology

    1.   Enucleated Superfused Rabbit Eye System
    2.   Balb/c 3T3 Cells/Morphological Assays (HTD)

B.  Cell Toxicity

    1.   Adhesion/Cell Proliferation

         a.   BHK Cells/Growth Inhibition
         b.   BHK Cells/Colony Formation Efficiency
         c.   BHK Cells/Cell Detachment
         d.   SIRC Cells/Colony Forming Assay
         e.   Balb/c 3T3 Cells/Total Protein
         f.   BCL-Dl Cells/Total Protein

    2.   Membrane Integrity

         a.   LS Cells/Dual Dye Staining
         b.   Thymocytes/Dual Fluorescent Dye Staining
         c.   LS Cells/Dual Dye Staining
         d.   RCE-SIRC-P815-YAC-1/Cr Release
         e.   L929 Cells/Cell Viability
         f.   Bovine Red Blood Cell/Hemolysis

    3.   Cell Metabolism

         a.   Rabbit Corneal Cell Cultures/Plasminogen Activator
         b.   LS Cells/ATP Assay
         c.   Balb/c 3T3 Cells/Uridine Uptake Inhibition Assay
         d.   Balb/c 3T3 Cells/Neutral Red Uptake
         e.   HeLa Cells/Metabolic Inhibition Test (MIT-24)

C.  Cell and Tissue Physiology

    1.   Epidermal Slice/Electrical Conductivity
    2.   Rabbit Ileum/Contraction Inhibition
    3.   Bovine Cornea/Corneal Opacity
    4.   Proptosed Mouse Eye/Permeability Test

D.  Inflammation/Immunity

    1.   Chorioallantoic Membrane (CAM)

         a.   CAM
         b.   HET-CAM
    2.   Bovine Corneal Cup Model/Leukocyte Chemotactic Factors
    3.   Rat Peritoneal Cells/Histamine Release
    4.   Rat Peritoneal Mast Cells/Serotonin Release
    5.   Rat Vaginal Explant/Prostaglandin Release
    6.   Bovine Eye Cup/Histamine (Hm) and Leukotriene C4 (LT-C4)
         Release

E.  Recovery/Repair

    1.   Rabbit Corneal Epithelial Cells/Wound Healing

F.  Other

    1.   EYTEX Assay
    2.   Computer Based/Structure Activity Relationship (SAR)
    3.   Tetrahymena/Motility

completely through an evaluation and the capital investment for facilities required to perform the test. The operational costs include technician time for maintenance of the test system and the biological component, professional time for evaluation of results, costs for non-biological components and technician time for endpoint analysis. Qualitative comments are given with respect to cost since it is generally impractical to attempt quantitative estimates at this stage.

The time required to conduct a particular test consists of 3 components: (a) the time to prepare stock cultures of the biological component in a format suitable for performing the test, (b) the actual time involved in the test procedure, and (c) the time for endpoint analysis. In each critique, the time commitment for each step in the process will be estimated. A rapid test is any test which can be completed within three days from the time the biological component is prepared and ready for test initiation to the completion of test data analysis.

TEST PROTOCOLS

The test systems which have been proposed as alternatives to the in vivo eye test can be classified on the basis of either the biological component (i.e. human corneal epithelial cell culture, bovine corneal explant culture, enucleated rabbit eyes, etc.) or on the basis of the endpoint measurement. We have selected the latter approach and have classified the alternative tests based on the nature of the endpoint measurement. To this end, we have utilized the classifications which are defined in the section on markers for test development (Chapter 5).

Studies which basically utilize morphological evaluations or observations which reflect gross morphological changes are included in the first group. The highest tolerated dose (HTD) assay developed by the Rockefeller group falls into this classification. Tests which measure corneal thickness also are classified in this group. Thus, the work of the Unilever group, the Shell U.K. group and the TNO-CIVO Institutes utilizing enucleated superfused rabbit eyes are discussed here.

The second collection of studies is classified as cell toxicity tests. The term cell toxicity, as used here, is taken in its more general interpretation to include not only cell lethality but also cellular dysfunction. This category can be further broken down into three subgroups: (1) adhesion/cell proliferation tests, (2) membrane integrity tests and (3) cell metabolism tests. Several tests which utilize colony formation efficiency and cell proliferation have been developed at the Institute of Toxicology in Zurich, Switzerland, Armour-Dial Inc., FRAME and the Rockefeller group and fall into the first subcategory. An equally large group of tests employ effects on membrane integrity to evaluate cytotoxicity. Dual dye staining techniques have been used by three different groups (at the University College of Wales, Johnson & Johnson, U.K. and the Institute of Toxicology, Zurich) while $^{51}$Cr release and red blood cell hemolysis has been studied at the University of Illinois and trypan blue staining at Hazleton Laboratories, Europe. Various aspects of cell metabolism have been investigated as a basis for toxicity evaluation, including protein synthesis (University of Washington and Tufts University), cellular ATP (University College of Wales), uridine uptake and neutral red uptake (Rockefeller group) and general cellular metabolism (University of Upsala). This latter subgroup of tests provides some insights into the effects of chemical agents on cellular functions.

Four tests have been identified which fall into the physiological response category. Studies of skin resistance (ICI) and the rabbit ileum system (Leicester Polytechnic) utilize physiological processes as the basis for toxicity evaluations. Tests which determine corneal opacity or corneal permeability have been developed at Leicester Polytechnic and Stanford University, respectively.

The next broad class of tests focuses on the problem of evaluating the inflammatory response. Studies utilizing the chorioallantoic membrane at Pennsylvania Medical College and the University of Munster have evaluated the inflammation responses in this tissue. Recent work at the University of Connecticut School of Medicine is investigating the release of mediators of the inflammatory response from the isolated bovine cornea. Other groups are evaluating the release of histamine (St. Johns University) and serotonin (Ortho Pharmaceutical Corp.) from peritoneal cells and both histamine and leukotriene C4 from bovine cornea. An approach at The Johns Hopkins University is investigating the release of prostaglandins by vaginal mucosal tissues. All of these tests are relevant to the inflammatory response of the eye.

The last classified group of tests involves those relating to repair/recovery. Currently only one proposed test has been adequately developed to address this important issue (Eye Research Institute). This is one area in which additional approaches are needed.

Finally, several tests did not fall into the proposed classification scheme. These include the computer based structure-activity relations developed at Health Designs, Inc., the EYTEX test developed at the National Testing Corporation and the Tetrahymena protozoan motility test (American Health Foundation). None of these tests has defined mechanistic basis directly related to the mammalian eye and thus cannot be classified by our system. However, they should be considered in any discussion of alternative approaches to eye toxicity testing.

In addition to the test protocols which have been classified above and are described in detail in the pages that follow, certain other avenues of research which are relevant to the issue of eye toxicology and testing should be noted. This work involves the broad area of endothelial cell culture studies. Many useful techniques have been developed over the years for evaluating the corneal endothelium in vitro. Cultured corneal endothelium has been used as an in vitro tool to evaluate substances anticipated to be injected into the anterior chamber of the eye during intraocular surgery. Dale Meyer, James McCulley and Michael Stern at the University of Texas have used this approach in defining the requirements of the corneal endothelium in terms of the ionic environment. Osmotic limits and pH also have been defined. The limits found in this system are similar to those found by Edelhauser (University of Milwaukee) in the whole corneal mount preparation. The composition of proposed formulations with the major active compound being a viscoelastic substance has been evaluated. This system has proved to be effective in determining the cytotoxicity or lack of cytotoxicity of proposed commercial viscoelastic preparations. Similar methods could be applied to the corneal epithelium which would relate more directly to alternatives to ocular irritancy tests.

The following are detailed descriptions of the specific alternative tests which have been proposed.

# A. Morphology

A.1.

GROUP: Morphology

TEST IDENTIFICATION: Enucleated Superfused Rabbit Eye System

I.  LOGISTICAL

   A.  Biological Component: Enucleated eyes from euthanized
   rabbits maintained in a superfusion system are utilized.

   B.  Non-Biological Component: A superfusion system which must be
   constructed by a mechanical shop (though not a very complex or
   expensive effort) is required. Constant temperature
   bath/circulating pump system and ophthalmascope are commercially
   available compounds of the system.

   C.  Endpoint Assay: Enucleated rabbit eyes are examined with a
   slit lamp before being used in a test and any eyes with
   abnormalities are rejected. At the same time the corneal
   thickness is measured using the Depth Measuring Attachment for the
   slit lamp. Repeated measurements are taken at the corneal apex
   and the scale on the depth-measuring device is read to the nearest
   0.01 units in the superfusion apparatus to ensure that the cornea
   had not been damaged during dissection. Two percent fluorescein
   sodium is applied to the surface of the cornea for a few seconds
   and then rinsed off with isotonic NaCl solution. Eyes that are
   significantly swollen after dissection, that stained with
   fluorescein or that showed any other signs of damage are rejected.

   The eyes are re-examined at intervals for up to 4 h after the
   application of the test substances and any changes in the normal
   appearance of the cornea are carefully noted. The corneal
   thickness also is measured and expressed either in terms of
   instrument units (1 unit = 0.8 mm) or as corneal swelling, which
   is expressed as [(corneal thickness at time t/corneal thickness
   before treatment) - 1] x 100%. The degree of swelling is used to
   grade the severity of response.

II. SCIENTIFIC

   A.  Endpoint Assay: This test system measures morphological
   alterations in an intact globe system. As such it is assumed that
   results will correlate linearly with results in the rabbit eye
   system while avoiding discomfort in animals. The endpoint is an
   objective measurement, but cannot be automated.

   B.  Correlation with Irritancy Data: The Unilever group has
   published a comparison of in vivo and in vitro results for 11
   identified compounds which shows good correlation between result
   generated by the test system and the reported in vivo irritancy
   classification. Equally good results were obtained by the Shell

group in a study investigating 60 unnamed chemicals.  Likewise, the TNO group reports 82% correlation for 32 unnamed chemicals. No direct comparisons with human data are provided.

III. ECONOMICS

The test system requires only a moderate amount of non-standard equipment and no great amount of technical expertise or time once operating.  Cost of compound evaluation should be less than that of the in vivo test system.  Additionally, an entire test should only take one day to perform.  This technology should be readily transferable.

IV.  COMMENTS

This test system shows promise as a screening system, but cannot be used to evaluate recovery and has the inherent variability of the basic in vivo system.  Perceived as an intact organ test system, yet (as currently performed) offers minimal advantages. The pursuit of measuring biochemical markers of inflammation in the system should be encouraged.  The majority of materials evaluated in this system to date have not been identified which makes the replication of results elsewhere difficult.

V.   REFERENCES

Burton, A.B.G., York, M. and Lawerence, R.S. (1981), The in vitro assessment of severe eye irritants, Fd. Cosmet. Toxicol, 19:471-480.

Koeter, H.B.W.M. and Prinsen, M.K. (1985), Introduction of an in vitro eye irritation test as a possible contribution to the reduction of the number of animals in toxicity testing.  CIVO Institutes TNO Report No. V 85.188/140322.

Price, J.B. and Andrews, I.J. (1985),  The in vitro assessment of eye irritation using isolated eye. Fd. Chem. Toxic, 23:313-480.

York, M., Lawerence, R.S. and Gibson, G.B. (1982),  An in vitro test for the assessment of eye irritancy in consumer products - preliminary findings. Int. J. Cosmetic. Sci., 4:223-234.

A.2.

GROUP:  Morphology

TEST IDENTIFICATION:        Balb/c 3T3 Cells/Morphological Assays (HTD)

I.   LOGISTICAL

A.    Biological Component:  The test system uses Balb/c 3T3 cells.

B.    Non-Biological Component:  Standard tissue culture
methodologies are employed in this test system.

C.    Endpoint Assay:  Balb/c 3T3 cells are seeded into 96 well
plates at a density that yields a semi-confluent culture 24 h
later.  At this time the media is removed and replaced with media
containing test chemical.  Cells are incubated in the presence of
the test chemical for 24 h at which point the cells are scored for
morphological alterations by phase contrast microscopy.  In a
second screening a narrower concentration range of toxicants is
tested.  The highest concentration of test chemical that does not
produce observable morphological alterations, relative to control
cells, is designated the highest tolerated dose (HTD).

II.  SCIENTIFIC

A.    Endpoint Assay:  This assay is based on a subjective
observation of morphological changes in cell structure using
normal controls in the same plate for comparison. The indices of
toxicity include a decrease in cell density and an increase in
cell rounding. An actual scoring for cytoplasmic abnormalities is
not necessary. The subjective endpoint has been verified, using
the more quantitative measurement of inhibition of colony
formation. It was found by comparing these two methods that the
HTD corresponded to the level of toxicant that reduced colony
formation to approximately 50%.  This study indicated that in the
hands of these investigators the subjective observation correlated
well with the quantitative observation. A collaborative study with
FRAME demonstrates that this test can be readily transferred to
other laboratories (personal communication).

B.    Correlation with Irritancy Data:  In one study the highest
tolerated dose assay was compared to the known ocular irritancy of
19 different chemicals.  There was an excellent correlation
between the test system and the known ocular effects of these
chemical. This study included ranking of chemicals for human
toxicity.

III. ECONOMICS

This assay utilizes standard tissue culture techniques for its
performance. The endpoint assay requires visual evaluation of
morphological changes in cells which can be rapidly (10-15 min per
plate) performed by low level technical personnel. This test can
be usefully employed as an preliminary range-finding test.

IV.  COMMENTS

In spite of the subjective nature of the endpoint measurement,
this test can be useful as a preliminary range-finding test as a

component of a complete test battery. The methodology can be readily transferred to other laboratories and does not require highly skilled technical personnel.

## V.    REFERENCES

Borenfreund, E. and Puerner, J.A.. (1984), A simple quantitative procedure using monolayer cultures for cytotoxicity assays (HTD/NR-90). J. Tissue Culture Methods, 9:7-10.

Borenfreund, E. and Puerner, J.A. (1985), toxicity determined in vitro by morphological alterations and neutral red absorption. Toxicol. Letters, 24:119-124.

Shopsis, C., Borenfreund, E., Walburg J. and Stark, D.M. (1985), A battery of potential alternatives to the Draize test: uridine uptake inhibition, morphological cytotoxicity, macrophage chemotaxis and expoliative cytology. F.D. Chem. Toxic, 23:259-266.

Borenfreund, E. and Shopsis, C. (1985), Toxicity monitored with a correlated set of cell-culture assays. Xenobiotica, 15:704-711.

# B. Cell Toxicity

## B.1. Cell Toxicity— Adhesion/Cell Proliferation

B.1.a.

GROUP: Cell Toxicity - Adhesion/Cell Proliferation

TEST IDENTIFICATION:  BHK Cells/Growth Inhibition

I.  LOGISTICAL

A.  Biological Component:  Baby Hamster Kidney Cells (BHK - 21 C13).

B.  Non-Biological Component:  Standard tissue culture methods and supplies.

C.  Endpoint Assay:  BHK cells are plated into 24 well culture plates (4 x $10^5$ cells per well) and incubated for 24 h.  The cells were washed and fresh medium containing test chemicals are added and cells exposed for 48 h.  The medium is discarded, the cells are washed with phosphate buffered saline and trypsinized for 5-15 min at $20^o$.  Fresh medium is added and cells are counted and expressed as a percentage of controls.  The lowest concentration of test chemical producing a significant inhibition of cell growth is determined ($GI_{Low}$).

II.  SCIENTIFIC

A.  Endpoint Assay:  This test measures a reduction in cell growth potential which can result from several factors, including cytotoxicity and retardation in cell division.  This assay endpoint is more sensitive than the cell detachment assay studied by this group (see BHK Cells/Cell Detachment).

B.  Correlation with Irritancy Data: Insufficient data are available for a meaningful evaluation of this test.

III.  ECONOMIC

This is a somewhat slow test system - 24 h preincubation, 48 h exposure to test chemical and several hours for cell counting and data analysis.  For automation a Coulter Counter is required.

IV.  COMMENTS

This test exhibits a high variability in the endpoint measured. The endpoint is subjective, unless automated, and the test takes considerable technical time.

V.   REFERENCES

Reinhardt, C.A., Pelli, D.A. and Zbinden, G. (1985), Interpretation of
cell toxicity data for the estimation of potential irritation.   Fd.
Chem. Toxic. 23:247-252.

B.1.b.

GROUP: Cell Toxicity -   Adhesion/Cell Proliferation

TEST IDENTIFICATION: BHK Cells/Colony Formation Efficiency

I.   LOGISTICAL

   A.   Biological Component:  Baby Hamster Kidney Cells (BHK - 21 C13).

   B.   Non-Biological Component:  Standard tissue culture methods and supplies.

   C.   Endpoint Assay:  BHK cells (100 cells/well) are distributed into 24 well plates containing media plus test chemical.  The cells are exposed to the test chemical for 7 days.  Cells are fixed and stained with Giemsa.  The lowest concentration of test chemical which significantly reduced cloning efficiency was determined ($CE_{Low}$).

II.  SCIENTIFIC

   A.   Endpoint Assay:  The cloning plating efficiency (CE) of cultured cells is influenced by many factors and thus a decrease in CE is an integrated response.  The investigators indicated that there was significant variability in CE with control values ranging from 15-35%.  The variability in CE was attributed to the stress involved in cell proliferation at very low cell densities (the lack of cell - cell interactions).

   B.   Correlation with Irritancy Data:  Insufficient data are available for a meaningful analysis.

III. ECONOMICS

   This is a slow assay - 7 day exposure to test chemical plus several hours for colony counting and data analysis.

IV.  COMMENTS

   This test may be useful as part of a test battery; however, it has a slow turnaround time and the problems with data variability may limit the usefulness of this assay.

V.   REFERENCES

Reinhardt, C.A., Pelli, D.A. and Zbinden, G.. (1985), Interpretation of cell toxicity data for the estimation of potential irritation.  Fd. Chem. Toxic. 23:247-252.

B.1.c.

GROUP: Cell Toxicity Adhesion/Cell Proliferation

TEST IDENTIFICATION:   BHK Cells/Cell Detachment

I.   LOGISTICAL

A.   Biological Component:  Baby Hamster Kidney Cells (BHK - 21 C13).

B.   Non - Biological Component:  Standard tissue culture methods and supplies.

C.   Endpoint Assay:  BHK cells are plated in 24-well plates ($10^4$ cells / $cm^2$ ) and allowed to settle and attach over 24 h.  The media is removed and replaced with fresh media containing the test chemical and incubated for 4 h.  The total number of cells plated is determined at the start of the experiment by trypsinization and counting of control wells.  Detached cells are counted and the concentration of test chemical producing a significant increase in cell detachment above controls ($CD_{Low}$) determined.  Maximum detachment in solvent controls was 5%.  Data are classified as Class I (Low) - $CD_{Low}$ > 500 mM, Class II (mild to moderate) - $CD_{Low}$ = 1-500 mM and Class III (strong) - $CD_{Low}$ <1 mM.

II.  SCIENTIFIC

A.   Endpoint Assay:  Cell detachment is an indication of either cell death or functional alteration in cellular attachment.  A comparison of BHK cells with 2 other cell types (Keller cells - human deploid fibroblast of skin origin and MRC -5 cells - human embryonic lung fibroblast) indicated that all 3 cell types gave similar test results.

B.   Correlation with Irritancy Data: Based on the classification of test chemicals as to human eye irritation given in Merck (1983) 25 out of 30 chemicals tested agreed with the human data.  The chemicals which were incorrectly classified included sodium hydroxide, zinc sulphate, allyl alcohol, 1-pentanol and ethanolamine.

III. ECONOMIC

This is a relatively fast assay - 24 h preincubation, 4 h exposure and several hours for cell counting and data analysis.  The cell counting can be automated using a Coulter Counter.

IV.  COMMENTS

If cell counting is performed manually this particular test may be difficult to quantitate and one might expect large variability.  Automation will improve significantly the usefulness of this test.

V.   REFERENCES

Reinhardt, C.A., Pelli, D.A. and Zbinden, G. (1985), Interpretation of cell toxicity data for the estimation of potential irritation. Fd. Chem. Toxic. 23:247-252.

B.1.d.

GROUP:  Cell Toxicity - Adhesion/Cell Proliferation

TEST IDENTIFICATION :  SIRC Cells/Colony Forming Assay


I.    LOGISTICAL

A.   Biological Component: SIRC cell line derived from normal
rabbit cornea (fibroblast-like).  These cells are available from
ATOC.

B.   Non-Biological Component: Standard tissue culture resources.

C.   Endpoint Assay:  The endpoint for this assay is cell colony
formation efficiency.  A fixed number (400) of SIRC cells are
plated on 60 mm culture dishes containing F12S media.  Cells are
incubated for 18 h at $37^{o}$ and the dishes are washed twice with F12
media.  Fresh media containing the test chemical are added to
triplicate/plates.  After 1 h of incubation at $37^{o}$ the dishes are
washed and incubated for 7 to 8 days with F12S media to allow
surviving cells to form visible colonies.  Colonies are fixed with
10% formalin and stained with 0.1% crystalline violet.  The
percent survival relative to the control plates are determined by
counting colonies with 10 or more cells.  The concentration of
test chemical giving 50% relative survival ($LC_{50}$) was determined
graphically using a probit analysis.

II.   SCIENTIFIC

A.   Nature of Endpoint: Basically this is a cytotoxicity test.
The number of colonies formed presumably represents the number of
surviving cell following exposure to the test chemical.  Reduced
colony formation efficiency also can be attributed to effects on
cell adhesion.

B.   Correlation with Irritancy Data:  The investigators performed
comparative studies using 13 surfactants representing 4 chemical
classes.  Rank correlation between $LC_{50}$ and Draize classification
was good (R=0.90). Two chemicals showed significant deviation -
possibly related to pH and/or molecular weight factors. The
authors state that results are consistent with "limited" human
data but specifics are not given. In a study of 6 shampoos the
rank correlation between this test and the Draize ranking was
perfect (R=1.0).

III.  ECONOMIC

The endpoint assay involving colony counting can be automated.
The length of time taken for the test involves 1 day for
preparation of cells and 7 to 8 days for cell incubation after
exposure to test chemical. One day will be required for colony
counting and data analyses, giving a total of 8 to 10 days for
completion of the test for 1 test chemical. Multiple test
chemicals can be evaluated simultaneously which  significantly
increases efficiency.  Facilities requirements include standard
tissue culture equipment.

IV.   COMMENTS

This test has a slower turn around time than many in vitro systems
and it may prove more difficult to quantitate reproducibly in
different laboratories due to the inherent variability of colony
formation efficiency.

V.    REFERENCES

North-Root, H., Yackovich, F., Demetrulias, J., Gacula, N. and Heinze,
J.E. (1982), Evaluation of an in vitro cell toxicity test using rabbit
corneal cells to predict the eye irritation potential of surfactants.
Toxicol. Letters. 14:207-212.

North-Root, H., Yackovich, F., Demetrulias, J., Gacula, N. and Heinze,
J.E. (1985), Prediction of the eye irritation potential of shampoos
using the in vitro SIRC toxicity test. Fd. Chem. Toxic. 23:271-273.

B.1.e.

GROUP:   Cell Toxicity - Adhesion/Cell Proliferation

TEST IDENTIFICATION:     Balb/c 3T3 Cells/Total Protein.

I.   LOGISTICAL

    A.   Biological Component:  Balb/c 3T3 cells.

    B.   Non-Biological Component:  Standard tissue culture
    methodologies.

    C.   Endpoint Assay:  Balb/c 3T3 cells are plated ($3 \times 10^3$ cells
    per well) into 96 well tissue culture test plates.  Twenty-four
    hours after plating, the media is removed and replaced with fresh
    media containing the test chemical.  Cells are cultured for 24 h
    in the presence of the test chemical at which point the media is
    removed and the cells washed. Sodium hydroxide (0.1N) is added to
    each well and the plates incubated for 15 min at $37^{\circ}$.  Next a
    diluted solution of Bio-Rad dye reagent is added to each well and
    the plates incubated for 30 min with agitation on a shaker.  The
    absorption of each well is then measured on a microplate reader at
    405 nm and 630 nm.  The absorption at 630 nm is corrected by the
    absorption at 405 nm to give the concentration of protein in ug
    protein/well.  A dose response curve is generated and the
    concentration of toxicant which causes a 50% decrease in total
    cell protein is determined.

II.   SCIENTIFIC

    A.   Endpoint Assay:  This test system basically measures the
    proliferation of cells in culture by assaying for total protein
    present in each well.   However, total protein also can be
    affected by effects on protein synthesis. This is an integrated
    measure of the effects of a toxicant on the cells and is
    quantitative and can be automated.

    B.   Correlation with Irritancy Data:  The test system has been
    evaluated using 9 shampoos, 6 surfactants and 6 metals as test
    chemicals. The results rank the test surfactants in the order of
    cationic greater than anionic greater than nonionic which agrees
    with data obtained by other in vitro test systems as well as
    rabbit eye irritancy testing.

III.   ECONOMICS

    This is a relatively simple test based on utilizing standard
    tissue culture techniques.  The endpoint assay can be automated
    and thus reduce technician time.  The total time for the assay
    requires 24 h for preparing the cells, 24 h for exposure to the
    test chemical and less than 1 h for the endpoint assay.  Because
    the system can be automated, many test chemicals can be tested
    simultaneously.

IV.   COMMENTS

    This test is potentially useful as part of a battery. It is simple
    and can be easily automated.

V.    REFERENCES

Shopsis, C.  and Eng, B. (1985), Rapid cytotoxicity testing using a
semi-automated protein determination on cultured cells. Toxicol.
Letters 26:1-8.

Stark, D.M., Borenfreund, E. Walberg, J. and Shopsis, C. (1985),
Comparison of several alternative assays for measuring potential
toxicants.  In, Alternative Methods in Toxicology, Vol. 3, A.M.
Goldberg (Ed.) Mary Ann Liebert, Inc., New York, 371-390.

B.1.f

GROUP: Cell Toxicity - Adhesion/Cell Proliferation

TEST IDENTIFICATION:  BCL-D1 Cells/Total Protein

I.  LOGISTICAL

 A.  Biological Component: BCL-D1 cells obtained from Gibco Ltd.

 B.  Non-Biological Component: Standard tissue culture methodologies.

 C.  Endpoint Assay: BCL-D1 cells maintained in BME Modified media containing 10% fetal calf serum, 1% non-essential amino acids, and 0.33 g/L kanamycin sulphate are plated at a density of $2 \times 10^{4}$ cells per well in 24-well plates. After 24 h the test chemical is added in fresh medium and the plates incubated an addition 72 h. At the end of the treatment period the cells are washed three times with phosphate-buffered saline (PBS) and fixed with 3% gluteraldehyde in PBS for 10-20 min. After removal of the fixitive, the cells are stained with Kenacid Blue stain solution for 30 min with gentle agitation. Unbound stain is removed by washing with ethanol:glacial acetic acid:water (10:5:85) until no visible blue color is present in the washings. Bound stain is extracted with a desorb solution consisting of 1M potassium acetate in 70% ethanol. After 15 min the dye concentration in the desorb solution is determined spectrophotometrically at 570 nm. The final measurement can be automated using a multi-well plate reader. The concentration of test chemical (ug/ml) which reduces the final total cellular protein by 20%, 50% and 80% when compared to controls is computed.

II.  SCIENTIFIC

 A.  Endpoint Assay: The total protein assay basically measures cell proliferation in culture. Total protein levels also can be affected by interference with protein synthesis. Therefore, this test system integrates the combined effects of the test chemical on several indices of toxicity. This endpoint assay is easily automated using readily available technology.

 B.  Correlation with Irritancy Data: This test system has been evaluated using 50 test chemicals in blind studies in several different laboratories under the coordination of FRAME. Most of the test chemicals selected for the FRAME validation study were not chosen because of their ocular irritation potential.

III. ECONOMICS

 This is a well documented test which basically uses a simple endpoint assay to evaluate effect of test chemicals on cell proliferation. The test utilizes standard cell culture techniques and is easily automated. The test take 24 h for establishment of cells in multi-well plates, 72 h for exposure to test chemical and less than 2 h for endpoint analysis.

IV.  COMMENTS

 This simple test is potentially useful as part of a test battery.

Its ultimate value must be established using a set of test
chemicals which are appropriate to the area of ocular irritation.

V.    REFRENCES

Balls, M. and Horner, S.A. (1985) The FRAME interlaboratory programme
on in vitro cytotoxicity. Fd. Chem. Toxic. 23:209-213.

Knox, P., Uphill, P.F., Fry, J.R., Benford, D.J. and Balls, M. (1986)
The FRAME multicenter project on in vitro cytotoxicity. Fd. Chem.
Toxic. (In Press).

# B.2. Cell Toxicity— Membrane Integrity

B.2.a.

GROUP:  Cell Toxicity - Membrane Integrity

TEST IDENTIFICATION:  LS Cells/Dual Dye Staining

I.  LOGISTICAL

A.  Biological Component:  LS cells, a suspension culture of L929 mouse fibroblast cells derived from murine areolar/adipose tissue. (Earlier studies utilized HEp 2 and HeLa cells derived from a human laryngeal and cervical carcinoma, respectively.)

B.  Non-Biological Component:  Standard tissue culture methods and supplies.

C.  Endpoint Assay:  Mouse LS cells ($0.9$-$1.0 \times 10^6$ cells) are placed in 25 ml siliconized flasks in a total volume of 5 ml of complete growth medium containing the test chemical.  During a 4 h exposure to the test chemical, cells are agitated in an orbital shaker bath (90 rev/min) at $37^\circ$ and gassed with 95% air/5% $CO_2$.  At the end of the exposure period an aliquot of the cell suspension is mixed with an equal volume of physiological solution containing 5 ug/ml fluorescein diacetate and 300 ug/ml ethidium bromide. Replicate samples are scored for green (live) versus red (dead) fluorescence.  Cell counting can be performed manually or automated.  The concentration of test chemical required to damage 50% of the cell population ($CD^{50}$) is determined following transformation of the data to a probit-log dose relationship and curve fitting by linear regression analysis.  Sodium dodecyl sulphate is included in each test as a positive control and the $CD^{50}$ for each test chemical is normalized by dividing by the $CD^{50}$ sodium dodecyl sulphate in the same test.  The normalized $CD^{50}$, denoted as NCD50, is reported.  Irritancy of a test chemical is classified as:  slight irritant, NCD 50 > 1 mg/ml, moderate irritant, NCD 50 = 0.7-0.85 mg/ml and severe irritant, NCD 50 < 0.6 mg/ml.

II.  SCIENTIFIC

A.  Endpoint Assay:  The dual fluorescent dye staining technique is basically a measure of membrane permeability which in turn reflects cell viability.

B.  Correlation with Irritancy Data:  The result of this test were compared with in vivo irritation results obtained specifically for this study by the CFR protocol.  Fifteen unspecified materials were tested and the results for the in vitro test compared favorably with the in vivo classification.  However, the selection of test materials did not include a large selection of moderately irritating substances in order to evaluate the resolving power of the test system.

III. ECONOMIC

The time of the test is 4 h for exposure to test chemical and several minutes to several hours for endpoint measurements and data analysis, depending on the degree of automation. The endpoint analysis requires at minimum a fluorescent microscope and for full automation an image analysis system (video/computer system).

IV.   COMMENTS

This test may be very useful as part of a battery; however, if automated then significant expense for equipment will be incurred. The lack of identification of chemicals makes replication and comparisons difficult.

V.    REFERENCES

Scaife, M.C. (1982), An investigation of detergent action on cells in vitro and possible correlations with in vivo data. Internat. J. Cosm. Sci. 4:179-193.

Scaife, M.C. (1985), An in vitro cytotoxicity test to predict the ocular irritation potential of detergents and detergent products. Fd. Chem. Toxic. 23:253-258.

B.2.b.

GROUP:   Cell Toxicity - Membrane Integrity

TEST IDENTIFICATION:   Thymocytes/Dual Fluorescent Dye Staining

I.   LOGISTICS

A.   Biological Component:   Freshly prepared, primary rat thymocyte cultures.

B.   Non-Biological Component:   Standard tissue culture methods and supplies.

C.   Endpoint Assay:   The assay is started by mixing 2.4 - 3.2 x $10^6$ thymocytes with a mixture of fluorescein diacetate and ethidium bromide in L-15 culture medium containing the test chemical.   Cells are simultaneously exposed and stained for 20 min and are evaluated by flow cytometry (at least $10^4$ cells are inspected).   In the optimum mode, forward light scattering is used to determine total cell count while fluorescence at 2 wavelengths, corresponding to the 2 dyes, is simultaneously measured.   The shift in the distribution of the fluorescent emission of fluorescein is used to evaluate cytoxicity.   The concentration of test chemical which produces a 25% shift in the peak maximum (FS 25) is the test endpoint.

II.   SCIENTIFIC

A.   Endpoint Assay:   Fluorescein diacetate penetrate the membrane of living cells and is hydrolyzed to fluorescein by intracellular enyzmes.   Fluorescein is retained intracellular as long as the plasma membrane remains intact.   Thus, live cells fluoresce green. Ethiduim bromide (EB) will only penetrate cells if the integrity of the plasma membrane has been compromised.   EB will penetrate the membrane following degenerative alterations and stain nuclear DNA with a red fluorescence.   Thus, dead cells stain red.   It is suggested that fluorescein retention rather than ethidium bromide exclusion is a more useful endpoint.

B.   Correlation with Irritancy Data:   12 test chemicals were evaluated.   In general, the cationic detergents were most toxic, followed by the anionic detergent (SDS) and by most of the nonionic detergents.   This is the same sequence as that for the known eye irritation potential of these detergents.   Two highly irritating chemicals (dimethylsulfate and allylalcohol) only give moderate cytotoxicity by this test suggesting that the primary effects of these 2 agents do not involve membrane damage directly.

III.   ECONOMICS

This test has 2 drawbacks from a practical point of view.   First, it requires preparation of primary cultures of thymocytes at the time the test is to be performed (this requires rats as cell donors and technicians trained in animal surgery).   Secondly, the endpoint assay requires the availability of a flow cytometer which is an expensive piece of equipment.

IV.   COMMENTS

This test requires freshly prepared thymocytes which involves animal surgery. It has been suggested (personal communication) that the test system will work for other types of cells in suspension culture, however, this has not yet been demonstrated. This test may be a very useful part of a battery but the equipment costs are significant.

V.    REFERENCES

Aeschbacher, M., Reinhardt, C.A. and Zbinden, G. (1986), A rapid cell membrane permeability test using fluorescent dyes and flow cytometry. In press Cell Biol. Toxicol.

B.2.c.

GROUP:   Cell Toxicity - Membrane Integrity

TEST IDENTIFICATION:   LS Cells/Dual Dye Staining

I.   LOGISTICAL

A.   Biological Component:   LS cells derived from NCTC L929 fibroblasts.

B.   Non-Biological Component:   Standard tissue culture resources and methods.

C.   Endpoint Assay:   LS cells are grown in 1 L round-bottomed flasks and maintained in suspension culture at $37^o$. Aliquots of $4.9 \times 10^6$ cells are placed in 25 ml Erlemeyer flasks and test chemicals added. Cells are incubated for 4 h under 95% air/5% $CO_2$ in an orbital incubator shaking at 90 rpm ($37^o$). An aliquot of the cell suspension is mixed with a solution of fluorescein diacetate and ethidium bromide. Esterase activity in living cells breaks down the fluorescein diacetate to fluorescein which fluoresces green. Dead cells will not break down and retain the substrate. Ethidium bromide will not penetrate intact cell membranes but rapidly stains nucleic acids with a red fluorescence in dead cells. Thus, green fluorescent cells are alive while red fluorescent cells are dead. Cells are counted under a fluorescence microscope in a silver-backed modified Fuchs - Rosenthal hemocytometer. Data are quantitated by determining the concentration of the test chemical resulting in 50% cell death $CD_{50}$).

II.   SCIENTIFIC

A.   Endpoint Assay:   The $CD^{50}$ assay based on fluorescent dye staining is a quantitative cytotoxicity assay. The test evaluates effects on both membrane integrity and intracellular esterase activity.

B.   Correlation with Irritancy Data:   There is limited data for correlating results with eye irritancy testing. The $CD^{50}$ is compared with the Draize classification of 11 unknown chemicals (rated: 4 mild, 3 moderate, 4 severe). Selecting an arbitrary cutoff limit for the $CD^{50}$ assay, the test correctly identified all mild, all severe irritants and 2 out of 3 moderates with 1 incorrectly classified as mild. The limited data give relatively good results.

III.   ECONOMIC

The test is rapid, involving a 4 h incubation followed by cell counting after staining. The endpoint can be automated but requires expensive equipment.

IV.   COMMENTS

The dual dye staining technique can be a very useful approach but is expensive to automate. The data presented are limited by lack of identification of chemicals which makes replication and comparison difficult.

V.    REFERENCES

Kemp, R.B., Meredith, R.W.J., Gamble, S. and Frost, M. (1983),  A rapid
cell culture technique for assaying the toxicity of detergent based
products in vitro as a possible screen for eye irritancy in vivo.
Cytobio. 36:153-159.

B.2.d.

GROUP:  Cell Toxicity - Membrane Integrity

TEST IDENTIFICATION:  RCE-SIRC-P815-YAC-1/$^{51}$Cr Release

I.  LOGISTICAL

   A.  Biological Component:  Four cell types were utilized in
   development of the test system.  Two continuous cell lines of
   murine origin (YAC-1 and P815) were selected because of their ease
   of handling and the fact that they are known to readily label with
   $^{51}$Cr.  Two adherent cell cultures were selected; SIRC because of
   its origin from rabbit corneal epithelial cells and its use in the
   colony formation assay of North-Root (SIRC Cells/Colony Forming
   Assay) and primary rabbit corneal epithelial cells to provide a
   comparison between primary cells and cell lines.

   B.  Non-Biological Components:  Standard tissue culture methods
   and supplies.

   C.  Endpoint Assay:  Cells are dispensed into 96 well microtiter
   plates (5 x 10$^4$ cells/well).  Adherent cells are labeled with $^{51}$Cr
   using 1000 uCi per 1 x 10$^7$ cells.  Cells were labeled for 18-24 h
   at which time the plates were washed and new media containing test
   chemical added.  Suspended cells were labeled with the same
   concentration of $^{51}$Cr but for only 2 h after which the cells were
   washed and dispensed into the microtiter plates at the
   concentration indicated above.  Cells were exposed to test
   chemical for time periods ranging from 0.5-4 h.  At the end of the
   exposure period the microtiter plates were centrifuged and the
   supernatants collected and counted in a gamma counter.  The test
   system is calibrated by measuring the $^{51}$Cr - release from cells
   cultured in media free from the test chemical and the $^{51}$Cr -
   release when cells were lysed with a commercial detergent.  To
   determine the concentration of test chemical which produces a
   cytotoxic response in 50% of the cells (CD$_{50}$), the actual counts
   in the supernatant of a test well is corrected by subtracting the
   number of counts released by cells incubated in normal media.
   This value is then expressed as a percentage of the maximum
   release by lysed cells.  A graphical representation of the data is
   generated by plotting this cytotoxicity value versus concentration
   of test chemical.  The CD$_{50}$ value is determined by linear
   interpolation of these curves.

II.  SCIENTIFIC

   A.  Endpoint Assay:  $^{51}$Cr-release is an objective measure of cell
   death.  There appears to be some problems with the reproducible
   labeling of cells since replicate assays on the same chemicals
   give significant variations in the CD$_{50}$ values.  This indicates
   that for the test to be useful it will require incorporation of a
   set of internal standards in each test run to adjust the
   calibration scale on a daily basis.

   B.  Correlation with Irritancy Data:  6 chemicals were tested for
   which data were available, using the reduced volume eye irritancy
   testing.  Five of the 6 test chemicals were correctly ranked.
   However, 1 chemical (Polysorbate 20) consistently produced
   significant cytotoxicity, yet is classified as non-irritating in
   vivo.  The mechanistic basis for this discrepancy is not known.

All cells utilized in this test gave consistently similar results with the suspended cells (P815 and YAC-1) being most sensitive and the SIRC cells showing the most variability. This last observation was attributed to a lack of uniform radiolabeling of the adherent cells.

III. ECONOMIC

This test utilizes standard tissue culture methodology. The time for the test involves 18-24 h for $^{51}$Cr labeling of the cells (2 h if suspension cells are used), 4 h for incubation with test chemicals and several additional hours for gamma counting and data analysis. This assay requires the availability of a gamma counter.

IV. COMMENTS

Although this test has an objective endpoint it requires the use of a gamma emitting radioactive isotope and the inherent problems associated with this use. The variability in labeling of cells with $^{51}$Cr is a considerable limitation.

V. REFERENCES

Shadduck, J.A., Everitt, J. and Bay, P. (1985), Use of in vitro cytotoxicity to rank ocular irritation of six surfactants. In, In Vitro Toxicology, A.M. Goldberg (Ed.), Alternative Methods in Toxicology, Vol. 3, Mary Ann Liebert, Inc., New York.

Douglas, H.J. and Spillman, S.D. (1983), In vitro ocular irritancy testing. In, Product Safety Evaluation, A.M. Goldberg (Ed.), Alternative Methods in Toxicology, Vol. 1, Mary Ann Liebert, Inc., New York, 205-230.

B.2.e.

GROUP:  Cell Toxicity - Membrane Integrity

TEST IDENTIFICATION:  L929 Cells/Cell Viability

I.   LOGISTICAL

A.   Biological Component:  L929 Cells, an established line of mouse embryo cells.

B.   Non-Biological Component:  Standard tissue culture methods and supplies.

C.   Endpoint Assay:  L929 cells ($7 \times 10^5$ cells/ plate) are placed in 60 mm plastic petri dishes  and pre-incubated for 18 h.  Test chemical dissolved in incubation media is added and cells exposed for 48 h.  Attached cells are trypsinized and combined with detached, floating cells.  The total number of viable cells were counted.  Straight lines are fitted to the data in the linear region of the dose-response curves by linear regression analysis. The endpoint is the concentration of test chemical which gives 100% mortality, i.e. the extrapolation of the linear regression curve to the dose-axis.

II.  SCIENTIFIC

A.   Endpoint Assay:  This is a straight forward cytotoxicity assay using 100% mortality as the endpoint.  This test system was proposed several years ago and reflects a relatively naive approach to quantitation of toxicity.

B.   Correlation with Irritancy Data:  The test system is evaluated using only 3 coded test chemicals which scored as high, moderate and low irritancy in the Draize eye test.  The test system clearly distinguished the most irritant test chemical from the least but could not differentiate between the moderate and high irritant.

III. ECONOMIC

This is a standard cell viability assay which takes 18 h for preincubation, 48 h for exposure and several hours for cell counting and data analysis.

IV.  COMMENTS

The published details are not adequate for an evaluation.

V.   REFERENCES

Simons, P.J. (1981),  An alternative to the Draize test.  In, The Use of Alternatives in Drug Research, A.N. Rowan and C.J. Stratmann, (Eds.), The MacMillan Press Ltd., London.

B.2.f

GROUP:     Cell Toxicity - Membrane Integrity

TEST IDENTIFICATION:   Bovine Red Blood Cell/Hemolysis

I.    LOGISTICAL

A.    Biological Component:  Erythrocytes obtained from bovine
venous blood.

B.    Nonbiological Components:  Standard tissue culture methods
and supplies.

C.    Endpoint Assay:  Bovine venous blood is collected in
Alsever's solution at a concentration of 10 ml of blood per 20 ml
of anticoagulant.  The blood is washed and the erythrocyte pellet
collected and suspended in phosphate-buffered saline or Eagle's
essential medium.  Red blood cells are diluted sufficiently so
that 100 ul placed in a flat bottom microtiter plate gives an
optical density reading of approximately 0.4 absorption units at
410 nm.  After the red blood cell suspension is appropriately
diluted, 100 ul volumes are dispensed in flat bottom microtiter
plates.  Serial twofold dilutions of test compounds are prepared
and 4 test wells are used for each dilution.  The negative control
is four wells given phosphate-buffered saline or Eagle's medium.
Positive wells contain 100 ul of sonicated erythrocyte solution
mixed with 100 ul of saline or Eagle's medium.  One hundred ul of
each dilution of each test material is dispensed per well.  The
plate is incubated in a humidified incubator at $37^{\circ}$ for 4 h.  At
the end of the incubation, the microtiter plates are centrifuged
at 10,000 rpm for 5 min, and 50 ul of the supernatant is
transferred to another 96 well flat bottom microtiter plates.
Endpoints are determined by use of an automated plate reader
operating at a wave length of 410 nm.  End points are expressed as
the cytotoxic dose 50% determined by simple linear interpolation.
The results also can be interpreted visually by observing
hemolysis or absence of hemolysis (presence of a pellet of
erythrocytes in the bottom of the well).

II.   SCIENTIFIC

A.    Endpoint Assay:  Hemolysis is an objective measurement of red
cell injury.[51] There are no problems related to prelabeling of the
cells as in Cr studies but care is required in handling
erythrocytes since they are subject to damage by contaminated
buffers, pH or osmotic shock.

B.    Correlation with Irritancy Data:  6 chemicals were tested for
which data were available, using the reduced volume rabbit eye
irritancy test.  Five of the 6 chemicals were correctly ranked.
One chemical (Polysorbate 20) consistently produced significant
cytotoxicity, yet is classified as nonirritating in vivo in
rabbits.  The mechanistic basis for this discrepancy is not known.
In contrast, Muir and coworkers tested hemolysis of bovine
erythrocytes using a phosphate-buffered saline solution and a
variety of surfactants.  The correlation of hemolytic activity in
vitro with rabbit eye irritation responses was poor (correlation
coefficients of approximately 0.3 to 0.4).

III.  ECONOMIC

The test uses a simple and inexpensive cell system.  Preparation time for collecting and washing the cells is 2 to 3 h.  Incubation time is 4 h and approximately 1 h is needed for evaluating hemolysis and calculating the data.  The test has not been done on erythrocytes older than 3 to 4 days, so a relatively reliable source of red blood cells is necessary.  The test may be adaptable to commercially available sheep red blood cells, but this has not been demonstrated.

IV.  COMMENTS

The test has an objective endpoint.  It does not require the use of radioactivity but does require the use of mammalian red blood cells.  It has not yet been tested on materials other than surfactants, and there are conflicting data on its utility with these materials.  Simplicity of this approach makes further development attractive.

V.  REFERENCES

Shadduck, J.P., Render, J., Everitt, J., Meccoli, R.A., and Essex-Sorlie, D. (in press) An approach to validation:  comparison of six materials in three tests.  In, In Vitro Toxicology - Approaches to Validation, A.M. Goldberg (Ed.) Alternative Methods in Toxicology, Vol. 5, Mary Ann Liebert, Inc., New York.

Muir, C.K., Flower, C., and Van Abbe, N.J. (1983) A novel approach to the search for in vitro alternatives to in vivo eye irritancy testing. Toxicology Letters 18,1-5.

# B.3. Cell Toxicity—Cell Metabolism

B.3.a

GROUP:  Cell Toxicity - Cell Metabolism

TEST IDENTIFICATION:  Rabbit Corneal Cell Cultures/Plasminogen
                      Activator

I.  LOGISTICAL

A.    Biological Component:  Cultured primary rabbit corneal
epithelial cells.

B.    Non-Biological Component:  Cell culture facilities and a
spectrophotometer.

C.    Endpoint Assay:  Corneal epithelium is isolated from
euthanized adult rabbits, then dissociated into single cells in
suspension.  Cells are plated and maintained until they grow to
confluence within 7 days.  The cells are exposed to test material
for less than 5 min, rinsed  and maintained in culture medium to
induce plasminogen activator secretion. After 2 days, plasminogen
activator level present in media is measured by a
spectrophotometric technique.  Decrease in plasminogen activator
level is expressed as a percentage inhibition of secretion
compared to control cells.

II.  SCIENTIFIC

A.    Endpoint Assay:  The endpoint measured in this test system is
a reduction in the appearance of a specific enzyme in the culture
medium. The mechanistic basis of this response is poorly defined
since many different factors potentially could contribute to the
observed effect.

B.    Correlation with Irritancy Data:  For the small data set
(eight identified materials) presented, the correlation with the
Draize scores is fair but not excellent.  Based on a poorly
characterized human data set for eight compounds, the test system
correctly identified three compounds as strong irritants, however,
sodium hypochlorite gave a strongly positive response in the test
system, yet is classified as nonhazardous to man.

III.  ECONOMICS

The test does not appear to be overly complicated or require
significant technician time so the test should cost less than the
in vivo test. Preparation of test cell cultures requires 7 days,
incubation of cells after exposure to test chemicals is for 2 days
and 1 day is required for endpoint assay and evaluation.

IV.   COMMENTS

The mechanistic basis for this test is not clear, although
inhibition of protein synthesis is a contributing factor. The data
on correlation  with other test system results is not yet adequate
for evaluation.

V.    REFERENCES

Chan, K.Y. (1985),  An in vitro alternative to the Draize test.  In, In
Vitro Toxicology, A.M. Goldberg (Ed.) Alternative Methods in
Toxicology, Vol. 3, Mary Ann Liebert, Inc., New York, 407-422.

Chan, K.Y., (1986 in press), Release of plasminogen activator by
cultured corneal epithelial cells during differentiation and wound
closure, Expt. Eye Res. 42.

Chan, K.Y., (1986 in press), Chemical injury to an in vitro ocular
system:  differential release of plasminogen activator.  Clin. Eye Res.
5.

B.3.b.

GROUP:  Cell Toxicity - Cell Metabolism

TEST IDENTIFICATION:    LS Cells/ATP Assay

I.  LOGISTICAL

    A.  Biological Component:  LS cells derived from NCTC L929
    Fibroblasts.

    B.  Non-Biological Component:  Standard tissue culture resources.

    C.  Endpoint Assay:  LS cells are grown in 1 L round-bottomed
    flasks and maintained in suspension culture at $37^{\circ}$.  Aliquots of
    $4.9 \times 10^6$ cells are placed in 25 ml Erleumeyer flasks and test
    chemical added.  Cells are incubated for 4 h under 95% air/ 5% $CO_2$
    in an orbital incubator shaking at 90 rpm ($37^{\circ}$).  After exposure
    to the test chemical, a sample of the cell culture is assayed for
    ATP content by the firefly luciferase bioluminescent reaction.
    Sodium lauryl sulfate is used as an internal standard.  Data are
    quantitated by determining the concentration of test chemical
    which produces a 50% reduction in cellular ATP levels from control
    level ($ATP_{50}$).

II.  SCIENTIFIC

    A.  Endpoints Assay: The $ATP_{50}$ assay measures the concentration
    of a critical cellular component thus reflecting disruption of
    cellular function.  This assay provides information about specific
    effects on cellular functions.  The ATP level is a potentially
    sensitive index because it reflects effects on the cell at a
    fundamental level.

    B.  Correlation with Irritancy Data:  There is limited data for
    correlating results with the Draize Test.  There was a significant
    inconsistency between the $CD_{50}$ determined by the LS cell/Dual Dye
    Staining and the $ATP_{50}$ assays for two of seven chemicals tested by
    both methods (cycloxheximide and 2,4-dinitrophenol).  In general,
    the data are insufficient to fully evaluate the test system.

III.  ECONOMIC

    The test is rapid - 4 h incubation followed by the ATP assay
    ($ATP_{50}$).  Standard cell culture procedures are utilized.  Full
    automation of the test system will be difficult.

IV.  COMMENTS

    The data to date are limited severely by lack of identification of
    chemicals which make replication and comparison difficult.

V.  REFERENCES

Kemp, R.B., Meredith, R.W.J. and Gamble, S. (1985), Toxicity of
commercial products on cells in suspension: a possible screen for the
Draize Eye Irritation Test. Fd. Chem. Toxic. 23:267-270.

B.3.c.

GROUP:  Cell Toxicity - Cell Metabolism

TEST IDENTIFICATION:  Balb/c 3T3 Cells/Uridine Uptake Inhibition Assay

I.   LOGISTICAL

A.   Biological Component:  Balb/c 3T3 cells.

B.   Non-Biological Component:  Standard tissue culture techniques.

C.   Endpoint Assay: Effects of chemicals are evaluated by the uridine uptake assay.  Cells are plated in 35 mm dishes at a density of 5 x10$^4$ per dish.  After 48 h the media is removed and fresh media containing the test chemical added.  Cells are exposed to the test chemical for 4 h at 37$^o$.  Media is removed and the cells are washed twice with Tris buffered saline.  Uridine uptake is determined during a 15 min incubation at 37$^o$.  Cells are then washed three times and lysed with sodium hydroxide.  An aliquot of lysate is analyzed for radioactive uridine by scintillation counting.  A second aliquot is analyzed for total protein. Results are expressed as a percentage of control uptake.  Relative toxicity of the test compound is established by determining the concentration of chemical  required to induce a 50% inhibition of uridine uptake (UI-50).  UI-50 values were calculated by linear regression analyses of data over a range of concentrations of test chemical.

II.  SCIENTIFIC

A.   Endpoint Assay: The endpoint measured, uridine uptake inhibition, provides information concerning the functional integrity of both the cellular membrane and uridine kinase enzyme system.  Alterations in either of these components of cellular function will be reflected in an inhibition of uridine uptake. Additional studies indicated that the endpoint is useful to investigate the reversible nature of intoxication. A recent development involving performance of the exposure to the test chemical in the absence of serum in the culture medium  appears to be a significant improvement.

B.   Correlation with Irritancy Data:  The investigator compared the UI-50 (50% inhibition of uridine uptake) with the Draize classification of 25 chemicals.  The only chemical significantly out of order was Triacetin which expressed a more severe effect in the test system than in eye irritancy testing.  It was suggested that this discrepancy was due to a trace contaminant in the test chemical.

III. ECONOMIC

This test utilizes a radioisotope $^3$H-uridine and the endpoint measurement requires scintillation counting.  Therefore the assay requires the availability of appropriate radiation detecting equipment.  The time for the test involves 48 h for preparation of cells, 4 h for exposure to test chemical and 15 min for the uridine uptake.  The analyses by liquid scintillation counting will require several additional hours for counting and data analyses.

IV. COMMENTS

Although this test has an objective endpoint, it requires the use of a radioactive isotope. This in itself is not a limiting factor, but the use of radioisotopes introduces logistical complications in laboratory proceedures.

V. REFERENCES

Shopsis, C. and Sathe. S. (1984), Uridine uptake inhibition as a cytotoxicity test: correlation with the Draize test. Toxicology 29:195-206.

Shopsis, C. (1984), Inhibition of uridine uptake and cultured cells: a rapid, sublethal cytotoxicity test. J. Tissue Culture Methods 9:19-22.

Shopsis, C., Borenfreund, E., Walberg, J. and Stark, D.M. (1985), A battery of potential alternatives to the Draize test: uridine uptake inhibition, morphological cytotoxicity, macrophage chemotaxis and exfoliative cytology. Fd. Chem. Toxic. 23:259-266.

B.3.d.

GROUP: Cell Toxicity - Cell Metabolism

TEST IDENTIFICATION: Balb/c 3T3 Cells/Neutral Red Uptake

I.    LOGISTICAL

      A.    Biological Component: Balb/c 3T3 mouse fibroblast cell lines. Cells are available from ATCC.

      B.    Non-Biological Component: Standard tissue culture methodologies.

      C.    Endpoint Assay: Stock cell cultures of 3T3 mouse fibroblasts are dissociated with 0.05% trypsin, 0.02% EDTA. To each well of a 96 well tissue culture microtiter test plate are seeded $9 \times 10^3$ cells and the plates incubated overnight at $37^\circ$. Culture media is removed and fresh media containing the test chemical is added to each well with four replicate wells per concentration and incubation is continued for 24 h. Control cultures, in 8 wells located in different areas of the plate, receive normal media without test agents. Benzalkonium chloride, at a concentration range of 0.5 to 6 ug/ml, serves as a positive control. At the end of the incubation period, media is removed and the cells are washed. A neutral red solution (50 ug/ml) prepared in media is added to each well and incubated for 3 h at $37^\circ$. The dye containing media is removed and cells are washed rapidly with 4% formaldehyde-1% $CaCl_2$ to remove unincorporated dye and to simultaneously promote adhesion of the cell to the substratum. The formaldehyde solution is removed and a mixture of 1% acetic acid-50% ethanol is added to extract the neutral red dye into solution. The absorbance of the extracted neutral red dye in solution is measured by an automated micro-titer plate reader. Results are expressed as a percentage of untreated control cultures and a complete toxicity curve generated.

II.    SCIENTIFIC

      A.    Endpoint Assay: This test system measures the uptake and accumulation of neutral red dye in the lysosomes of living cells. It is not know whether this process requires active transport, however, the retention of the dye in the cells requires that the membranes be relatively intact. This is a quantitative endpoint which is amendable to automation.

      B.    Correlation with Irritancy Data: The investigators make a direct comparison between the neutral red assay and eye irritancy testing, and with the highest tolerated dose assay (HTD assay). The correlation with a limited number of compounds is encouraging.

III. ECONOMICS

      The test system utilizes standard tissue culture techniques. The endpoint assay can be automated and this will result in a reduction in technician time.

IV.    COMMENTS

      This test is a potentially useful part of a battery. The endpoint measurement uses a vital stain which provides information on the health of the cell rather than its ill health.

## V.    REFERENCES

Borenfreund E. and Puerner, J.A.  (1984), A simple quantitative procedure used in monolayer cultures for cytotoxicity tests. J. Tissue Culture Meth. $\underline{9}$:7-10.

Borenfreund, E. and Puerner, J.A. (1985), Toxicity determined in vitro by morphological alterations and neutral red absorption. Toxicol. Lett. $\underline{24}$:119-124.

Shopsis, C. and Borenfreund, E., (1985), In vitro cytotoxicity assays: Potential alternatives to the Draize test.  In, Evaluation Des Effects Cosmetiques Methodes D'Aujourd'Hui et de Demain.  Proceeding of XVemes Journees Internationales de Dermocosmetologie de Lyon, June 5, 6, 7, 1985.

B.3.e.

GROUP:  Cell Toxicity - Cell Metabolism

TEST IDENTIFICATION: HeLa Cells/Metabolic Inhibition Test (MIT-24)

I.  LOGISTICAL

A.  Biological Component:  HeLa cells.

B.  Non-Biological Components: Standard tissue culture methods and supplies.

C.  Endpoint Assay:  HeLa cells are continuously subcultured in Parker 199 medium supplemented with 10% v/v calf serum.  Before use in test, the cells are harvested using Versene (0.2 mg EDTA /L PBS) and made round by suspension in a spinner culture for 2 h. Test chemical in Parker 199 medium is added to the appropriate wells of a 96 flat-bottom well, microtitre plate and $1 \times 10^{4}$ cells are added to each well.  The final test media consisted of Parker 199 medium supplemented with 5% v/v calf serum, 3 mg/ml glucose, 20 mg/ml phenol red, 200 i.u./ml benzylpenicillin, 0.1 mg/ml streptomycin sulphate and varying concentration of test chemical. Cultures were sealed with sterile liquid paraffin and plastic film and incubated at $37^{\circ}$ for 24 h (the original test called for a 7 day incubation).  At the end of the test the pH of each culture well is  determined by observation of the color of the phenol red in the medium.  Violet cultures (pH > 8.0) are considered totally inhibited, orange-yellow cultures (pH 6.0 - 6.5) are considered totally viable (acid pH indicates the production of acid metabolites by cells), and red cultures are considered partially inhibited.  Approximate IC 50 values (50% inhibitory concentration) are calculated as the geometrical mean value between the  minimal total inhibitory and the maximal non-inhibitory concentrations.

II.  SCIENTIFIC

A.  Endpoint Assay:  Measurement of the pH change in a closed culture system is a simple though crude technique to determine whether cells retain some degree of metabolic competence following exposure to a test chemical.  The endpoint can be quantitated although the current test uses a visual subjective judgment of color.

B.  Correlation with Irritancy Data:  The results of the MIT-24 test and Draize classification for 18 chemicals are given. Although the authors discuss only 2 out of 18 chemicals as incorrectly ranked (1-heptanol and allyl alcohol) there appear to be several others which are classified by the MIT-24 test to be more cytotoxic than is suggested by in vivo ranking (sodium lauryl sulphate, trichloroacetic acid, Solketol and isopropyl alcohol). Thus, approximately one third of the chemicals tested are incorrectly ranked.

III.  ECONOMICS

This is an extremely simple and relatively rapid test.  The techniques employed are standard tissue culture procedures and the endpoint requires no equipment for quantitation.

IV.    COMMENTS

The assumptions underlying this test have to be defined before a realistic evaluation can be obtained.  The test agent can, for example, affect pH alone and that would produce aberrant results. Further, the assumption is made that metabolism and viability are linearly related. These questions have not been critically investigated.

V.    REFERENCES

Selling, J. and Ekwall, B. (1985),  Screening for eye irritancy using cultured HeLa cells. Xenobiotica 15:713-717.

# C. Cell and Tissue Physiology

C.1.

GROUP: Cell and Tissue Physiology

TEST IDENTIFICATION:     Epidermal Slice/Electrical Conductivity

I.   LOGISTICAL

    A.   Biological Component:  Skin slices from rats obtained
    following humane sacrifice.

    B.   Non-Biological Component:  Standard organ techniques.  A
    simple apparatus to mount the tissue must be constructed.

    C.   Endpoint Assay: Epidermal skin slices obtained from albino
    Wistar rats are mounted on a plastic tube and the electrical
    resistance across the skin slice is measured using a standard
    electrical resistance circuit.  A positive result for a test
    chemical is determined when the electrical resistance decreases
    below 4K ohm after 24 h of exposure to the test chemical.

II.  SCIENTIFIC

    A.   Endpoint Assay: The electrical resistance is a measure of the
    integrity of the stratum corneum/epidermis.  The relationship
    between electrical resistance and membrane integrity was verified
    by demonstrating a correlation between electrical resistance and
    water permeability of the skin slices as measured by $^3$H-water
    penetration through the skin slices.

    B.   Correlation with Irritancy Data: Out of 41 human skin
    corrosive agents all but 4 were correctly identified (less than
    10% false negatives).  Of 22 irritants, 8 were positive in the
    test (false positives) which were all surfactants.

III. ECONOMICS

    This method utilizes animals as skin donors and multiple test can
    be performed from one animal.   This is a economical use of animal
    resources. The test time is 24 h with little additional time for
    analyses.

IV.  COMMENT

    Although this test is for identifying corrosive chemicals, its
    relevance to eye testing is that all agents which are positive as
    skin corrosives can be assumed to be severe eye irritants and thus
    eliminate eye testing.

V.   REFERENCES

Oliver, C.J.A., and Pemberton, N.A. (1985), An in vitro epidermal slice
technique for identifying chemicals with potential for severe cutaneous
effects. Fd. Chem. Toxic. 23:229-232.

C.2.

GROUP:   Cell and Tissue Physiology

TEST IDENTIFICATION:      Rabbit Ileum/Contraction Inhibition

I. LOGISTICAL

   A.   Biological Component: Isolated segments of the rabbit
   terminal ileum.

   B.   Non-Biological Component:  An isolated organ bath system.

   C.   Endpoint Assay:  Segments of the terminal ileum of California
   white rabbits are isolated and mounted in an organ bath under a
   tension of 1.0 g.  The tissue is bathed in Tyrode Ringer solution
   at $35^{o}$ and bubbled with air.  Spontaneous contractions are
   recorded using isotonic transducers and an oscilloscope.  The
   tissue is allowed to equilibrate for 25 min before test chemicals
   are added.  Aliquots of test chemical are added at 10 min
   intervals until the spontaneous activity level is reduced to 50%
   of the control level (EC 50).  If greater than 50% inhibition of
   spontaneous activity is not achieved after 5 additions the tissue
   is discarded.

II.   SCIENTIFIC

   A.   Endpoint Assay:  The rationale for this test is that it
   evaluates both the ability of the test chemical to penetrate
   several cellular layers as well as its ability to interfere with
   cellular function (muscle contraction).  It is not clear how the
   effects on muscle contraction, which could involve electrochemical
   as well as mechanical processes, relate to cellular injury which
   produces eye damage.

   B.   Correlation with Irritancy Data: In one study the in vitro
   test was compared to in vivo data for 8 surfactants.  There was
   reasonable agreement between the two sets of data for the least
   irritating chemicals but there was considerable disagreement on
   the ranking of the most highly irritating test chemical.  A second
   study made a similar comparison of 12 chemicals, using the in vivo
   data of Carpenter and Smyth (Am. J. Ophthalmol. 29:1363-1372,
   1946). Here the in vitro test selected the least and most
   irritating test chemicals but disagreed on ranking of intermediate
   strength chemicals.  The investigator attributes the discrepancies
   to the imprecise nature of the in vivo data.

III. ECONOMICS

   This test system requires a physiological apparatus for mounting
   and measuring the excised ileum as well as animal surgical
   expertise.  It is not clear from the literature exactly how many
   viable ileum segments can be obtained from one rabbit on average.

IV.  COMMENTS

   Although proposed as an alternative to in vivo eye irritancy
   testing extensive assumptions must be accepted which limits the
   interpretability of the data.  To date, the correlation is poor.

V.    REFERENCES

Muir, C.K., Flower, C., and Van Abbe, N.J., (1986), The effect of shampoos on rabbit ileum in vitro compared to eye irritancy in vivo. J. Am. College of Tox. 5:2,113.

Muir, C.K., Flower, C. and Van Abbe, N.J. (1983),  A novel approach to the search for in vitro alternatives to in vivo eye irritancy testing. Toxicol. Let. 18:1-5

Muir, C.K. (1983), The toxic effect of some industrial chemicals on rabbit ileum in vitro compared with eye irritancy in vivo. Toxicol. Let. 19:309-312.

C.3.

GROUP:  Cell or Tissue Physiology

TEST IDENTIFICATIONS:  Bovine Cornea/Corneal Opacity

I.   LOGISTICAL

A.   Biological Component:  Isolated bovine cornea obtained from a slaughterhouse.

B.   Non-Biological Component:  A specially designed cell which fits into an opacitometer.  This equipment is designed and fabricated by the investigator and is not available commercially.

C.   Endpoint Assay:  Freshly isolated bovine cornea are mounted in a perspex holder and bathed with Tyrode solution on both sides. The test chemical is added to the component bathing either the epithelial or endothelial side of the corneal tissue.  The holder is placed in the opacitometer which is zeroed using a blank holder in the chamber.  The transmission of white light through the cornea is measured as a function of time; increasing opacity being indicated by a drop in the voltage across the photocell. Immediately prior to a measurement in the photocell the culture media is replaced with fresh Tyrode solution to eliminate turbidity in the bathing solution as a confounding factor. Incubation in the presence of test chemical are carried out at $32^{o}$ for up to 6 h.  Concentration - opacity curves are constructed for experimental data at 6 h.  No standard classification scale is reported.

II.  SCIENTIFIC

A.   Endpoint Assay:  The test system evaluates the development of corneal opacity during exposure to test chemicals.  This effect reflects both physiological and gross morphological changes in the corneal structure.  The system described allows for a quantitative, objective measurement of this phonomena.

B.   Correlation with Irritancy Data:  Data for a total of 13 test chemicals are reported (5 anionic surfactants 3 cationic surfactants and 5 industrial chemicals).  For the eight surfactants a correlation coefficient of 0.854 was obtained by comparing the opacity produced at a $10^{-2}$ M concentration of the test chemical with in vitro ocular toxicity.  For the five industrial chemicals tested, the in vitro test gave the identical order for the opacity as was observed in vivo when the data at a test concentration of 10% v/v were used.  The results were less well differentiated at lower concentrations of test chemical.  In general this test reflected the in vivo data rather well, however, different concentration of test chemicals were used for the different chemical classes when comparisons were made to in vivo data.  This lack of standardization of the endpoint classification must be resolved.

III. LOGISTICAL

The test system requires the availability of bovine cornea from a slaughterhouse and the construction of a rather simple apparatus for test measurements.  The test is rapid but requires a technician with surgical skills.

IV.   COMMENTS

This test utilizes a quantitative endpoint which may be difficult
to intrepret.  It uses tissues from animals which will be
sacrificed for other purposes.  The main drawback at this time is
that the endpoint measurement must be standardized and a
classification scale developed which can be used to evaluate
toxicity in a systematic manner.

V.    REFERENCES

Muir, C.K. (1984), A single method to assess surfactant-induced bovine
corneal opacity in vitro: Preliminary findings.  Toxicol. Let.
22:199-203.

Muir, C.K. (1985), Opacity of bovine cornea in vitro induced by
surfactants and industrial chemicals compared with ocular irritancy in
vivo. Toxicol. Let. 24:157-162

C.4.

GROUP:  Morphology and Physiology

TEST IDENTIFICATION:  Proptosed Mouse Eye/Permeability Test

I.   LOGISTICAL

A.   Biological Component:  Eyes of freshly killed mice.

B.   Non-biological Component:  A specially designed
fluorophotometer.

C.   Endpoint Assay:  The mouse is asphyxiated in $CO_2$, the eyes
are proptosed in situ and the corneas are exposed to a drop of
toxicant for 1 min.  In the test as originally described, one eye
was used as a control for the other, but it has proved more
efficient to use each eye for a separate test material.  The eyes
are washed and then exposed to a drop of sulforhodamine B for
1 min and washed again.  The fluorescence of the cornea resulting
from the penetration of the dye is then measured.  About 10 levels
of acquired fluorescence can be meaningfully distinguished.

II.  SCIENTIFIC

A.   Endpoint Assay:  The test system measures the permeability
change in the epithelial barrier after exposure to test
substances.  It is a sensitive technique for quantitating the
integrity of the epithelial barrier.

B.   Correlation with Irritancy Data:  The test system seems to
correlate reasonably well with the two compounds tested.  Sodium
hydroxide and benzalkonium chloride gave graded increases in the
penetration value as their concentrations rose; the rise in index
corresponds roughly to the injury caused to the living eye.

III. ECONOMICS

This is a relatively simple test that can be learned easily.  The
cost of mice and their housing is minimal.  Many substances can be
tested in an hour, and the results are immediately available.
Currently available fluorometers are expensive and not suitable
for the purpose.  An instrument has been designed specifically for
the test, which would cost about $1,000 to fabricate on an
individual basis.

IV.  COMMENTS

This is a straightforward test that has the drawback that mice
must be freshly killed; however, it avoids discomfort to living
animals.  It has economic advantages that may make it valuable as
part of a battery of screening tests.  However, its utility is not
yet proven with a wide range of test chemicals.

V.   REFERENCES

Brooks, D. and Maurice, D.  A simple fluorometer for use with a
permeability screen.  Alternatives to Animal Testing, Vol. 5., In
press.

# D. Inflammation/Immunity

## D.1. Chorioallantoic Membrane (CAM)

D.1.a.

GROUP:  Inflammation/Immunity

TEST IDENTIFICATION: CAM (Chorioallantoic Membrane)

I.   LOGISTICAL

   A.   Biological Component:  The chorioallantoic membrane of chick embryo.

   B.   Non-Biological Component:  Standard equipment to incubate and examine chicken eggs, plus a standard microscope.

   C.   Endpoint Assay:  Fertile eggs, day 0, are incubated at $37^\circ$. On day 3 of incubation the shell is penetrated in two places. First, near the pointed end of the egg a small opening is ground in the shell and the shell membrane is exposed.  With a shortened needle and syringe the shell membrane is penetrated and 1.5 to 2 ml of albumin is removed and discarded.  The second opening is a rectangular window.  The window is closed with transparent tape until the next step.  On day 14 the tape is removed, opening the window.  A Teflon ring, 10 mm in internal diameter, is placed on the CAM (chorioallantoic membrane). The ring serves as a marker of the test site and as a container for the preparation to be tested. An aliquot of the test sample is placed in the ring, using an Eppendorf pipette.  The window is closed again with tape and the egg returned to the incubator.  Three days later, on day 17 of incubation, the tape is removed and the CAM examined.  The criteria used for macroscopic rating of lesions on the chorioallantoic membrane are listed below:

   a. Size
   b. Contours and surface
        Raised, flat, or depressed
        Edges raised
        Smooth, granular or shaggy
        Transparent or opaque
   c. Color
        White, yellow, red, brown, grey or black
   d. Retraction of surrounding CAM
   e. Spokewheel pattern of vessels
   f. Overall grade of severity
   g. Necrosis (confirmed microscopically)

II.  SCIENTIFIC

A.  Endpoint Assay:  The test system evaluates inflammation in the tissue system utilized in a subjective manner.  The mechanistic relationship between CAM and human ocular responses is not clear.  There is a noticeable variability in response between individual eggs.

B.  Correlation with Irritancy Data: Results for 12 unnamed materials have been reported and a rank correlation of 0.72 was observed.

III.  ECONOMICS

The large number of eggs needed per test (60) overcomes the relatively low cost of the model system and low labor costs per single test unit.  Cost should be comparable to the rabbit in vivo test.  The procedure requires that the eggs be prepared 2 weeks prior to the test, three days for exposure to the test chemical and less than 1 h for grading. If microscopic confirmation is required, significant additional time is needed for preparation of sections.

IV.  COMMENTS

The system is simple, but the overall usefulness is not yet fully defined.  Significant effort by a number of different laboratories needs to be performed to address the large questions of subjectivity, reproducibility and correlation with results in rabbits and humans. Recent studies in two different laboratories (Lawrence et al. 1986; Price, et al. 1986), using test systems similar to the one described here, indicated only moderate correlations with Draize scores.

V.  REFERENCES

Leighton, J., Nassauer, J. and Tchao, R. (1985),  The chick embryo in toxicology:  an alternative to the rabbit eye, Fd. Chem. Toxic., 23:291-298.

Leighton, J., Nassauer, J., Tchao, R. and Verdone, J. (1983), Development of a procedure using the chick egg as an alternative to the Draize rabbit test. In, Product Safety Evaluation A.M. Goldberg (Ed.), Alternative Methods in Toxicology, Vol. 1, Mary Ann Liebert, Inc., New York, 165-177.

Leighton, J., Tchao, R., Verdone, J. and Nassauer, J. (1985), Macroscopic assay of focal injury in the charioallantoic membrane.  In, In Vitro Toxicology A.M. Goldberg (Ed.), Alternative Methods in Toxicology, Vol. 3, Mary Ann Liebert, Inc., New York, 357-370.

McCormick, J.F., Nassauer, J., Bielunas J. and Leighton, J. (1984), Anatomy of the chick charioallantoic membrane relevant to its use as a substrate.  In Bioassay Systems.  Scanning Electron Microscopy IV, 2023-2030.

Lawrence, R.S., Groom, M.H., Ackroyd, D.M. and Parish, W.E. (1986), The chorioallantoic membrane in irritation testing. In press, Food Chem. Toxicol.

Price, J.B., Barry, M.P. and Andrews, I.J. (1986), The use of chick chorioallantoic membrane to predict eye irritants. In press, Food Chem. Toxicol.

Kong, B.M., Viau, C.J., Rizvi, P.Y. and DeSalva, S.J. (in press). The development and evaluation of the chorioallantoic membrane (CAM) assay. In, In Vitro Toxicology - Approaches to Validation, A.M. Goldberg (Ed.), Alternative Methods in Toxicology, Volume 5, Mary Ann Liebert, Inc., New York.

D.1.b

GROUP: Inflammation/Immunity

TEST IDENTIFICATION: HET-CAM

I.   LOGISTICAL

    A.   Biological Component: The natural chorioallantoic membrane of the chick embryo (day 10).

    B.   Non-biological Component: Standard equipment to incubate and examine chicken eggs.

    C.   Endpoint assay: Fertile eggs, day 0, are incubated at $37.5^{o}$ ($\pm 0.5^{o}$) at a relative humidity of 65% ($\pm 10$%). On day 10, the egg shell of 6 eggs per test is scratched around the air cell; the shell and the inner egg membrane are removed and the natural CAM is laid open for examination; 0.2 - 0.3 ml of liquid or 0.1 g of solid test sample are placed on the CAM and the reactions are observed, scored and classified over a 5 min period as follows:

Scoring Scheme for Irritation Testing with the HET-CAM

| | | Score | | |
|---|---|---|---|---|
| Effect | Time (min)... | 0.5 | 2 | 5 |
| Hyperaemia | | 5 | 3 | 1 |
| Haemorrhage | | 7 | 5 | 3 |
| Coagulation | | 9 | 7 | 5 |

Classification of Cumulative Scores in the HET-CAM

| Cumulative Score | Irritation Assessment |
|---|---|
| 0-0.9 | Practically None |
| 1-4.9 | Slight |
| 5-8.9 | Moderate |
| 9-21 | Strong |

II.  SCIENTIFIC

    A.   Endpoint Assay: The test system measures inflammation (hyperaemia), hemorrhages and corrosiveness (coagulation). The natural CAM is a vital and vascularized membrane; however, the relation to responses in tissues is not well defined.

    B.   Correlation with Irritancy Data: The University of Muenster group has reported positive correlations on a limited database.

III. ECONOMICS

    The costs of the model system, per the single test unit and labor costs are relatively low and may be lower than for the rabbit eye test. After 10 day incubation of fertile eggs, the CAM is exposed

to test chemical, examined, and test results classified, a
procedure that requires only 5 min.

IV.   COMMENTS

The test system is simple and relatively inexpensive, however the
ultimate value is yet to be determined. A 2-year validation study
in the Federal Republic of Germany is in progress and the results
of this project should be useful in evaluating the HET-CAM test.

V.   REFERENCES

Luepke, N.P. (1985), Hen's egg chorioallantoic membrane test for
irritation potential, Fd. Chem. Toxic. 23:287-291.

Luepke, N.P. (1985), HET - Chorioallantoic test:  An alternative to the
Draize rabbit eye test.  In, In Vitro Toxicology A.M. Goldberg (Ed.),
Alternative Methods in Toxicology, Vol. 3, Mary Ann Liebert, Inc., New
York, 591-606.

D.2.

GROUP: Inflammation/Immunity

TEST IDENTIFICATION:     Bovine Corneal Cup Model/Leukocyte Chemotactic
                         Factors

I.  LOGISTICAL

    A.   Biological component:  Isolated bovine corneas obtained from a
slaughterhouse.

    B.   Non-Biological Component:  Paraffin cup mount.

    C.   Endpoint Assay:  Isolated corneas are maintained in cold,
phosphate buffered saline (pH 7.3) until used.  The tissue is
mounted in a paraffin well with the epithelial surface facing
upwards and both surfaces are bathed in serum-free Minimal
Essential Media.  The epithelial surface is treated with the test
chemical for a period of time which varies depending on the test
chemical used.  The test chemical is removed by washing and
replaced with fresh media.  The corneas are incubated for up to
6 h.  Samples of the media in contact with the epithelial surface
are removed and assayed for chemotactic activity in a modified
Boyden Chamber.  Neutrophils and mononuclear cells isolated from
fresh bovine blood are used as indicator cells.  Penetration of
indicator cells into a micropore membrane is determined and test
results are presented as a percentage of the response to a positive
control ($C_5$ fragment).  A quantitative endpoint calibration scale
has not been established, thus chemicals are merely ranked relative
to each other.

II.  SCIENTIFIC

    A.   Endpoint Assay:  The test system is designed to evaluate the
release of chemotactic factors by corneal tissues in culture.
These factors act as mediators in the inflammatory process and thus
chemically induced release of such factors could play a fundamental
role in the development of ocular pathology.  The assay for
chemotactic factors, using leukocyte migration in a Boyden Chamber,
is a difficult, time consuming assay which requires the preparation
of indicator cells.

    B.   Correlation with Irritancy Data: This test system is in its
initial development stage and as such insufficient data are
available for evaluating its potential for eye irritation and
inflammation testing.  Preliminary studies utilizing hydrogen
peroxide and sodium hydroxide have been undertaken.

III.  ECONOMIC

This test system utilizes bovine cornea which are obtained fresh
from a local slaughterhouse.  Such material may not be universally
available.  The endpoint assay as currently performed requires the
preparation of indicator cells for the chemotactic factor assay.
The procedures employed for preparation of indicator cells require
trained technical assistance as well as bovine blood.  The test
protocol can be completed in one day, however, there is significant
personnel time invested.  At the present time this endpoint assay
cannot be automated.

IV.   COMMENTS

This test system has significant potential for providing important information concerning the inflammatory component of ocular toxicity.  The test protocol requires significant development in terms of standardization of a test protocol and a calibration scale which can be used to classify the response to chemical agents.  A major improvement of the test system awaits the development of an Elisa assay for the specific chemotactic factors, however, with such development the assay can be automated.

V.   REFERENCES

Elgebaly, S.A., Herkert, N., O'Rourke, J. and Kreutzer, D.L. (1986), Characterization of neutrophil and monocyte specific chemotactic factors derived from the cornea in response to hydrogen peroxide injury. Submitted for publication.

Elgebaly, S.A., Downes, R.T., Foronhar, F., O'Rourke, J. and Kreutzer, D.L. (1986), Inflammatory mediators in alkali-burned corneas: Inhibitory effects of citric acid.  Submitted for publication.

D.3.

GROUP:  Inflammation/Immunity

TEST IDENTIFICATION:  Rat Peritoneal Cells/Histamine Release

I.   LOGISTICAL

A.   Biological Component:  Rat peritoneal cells obtained by
peritoneal lavage following humane sacrifice.

B.   Non-Biological Component:  Standard tissue culture methods and
supplies.

C.   Endpoint Assay:  Rat peritoneal cells, including 4-6% mast
cells, are obtained by peritoneal lavage.  Several rats are
required for a dose response study and all cells were pooled to
reduce inter-animal variability.  Harvested cells are maintained at
$4^{\circ}$ throughout isolation and suspended in Hanks's balanced salt
solution containing 10% bovine serum albumin until used in the
test.  Cells are exposed to the test chemical at $39^{\circ}$ for 10 min
using 5 replicates at each test concentration.  Exposure was
terminated by the addition of ice cold 0.9% NaCl.  Cells are
pelleted (400g - 10 min) and supernatant collected and stored at -
$15^{\circ}$ until assayed.  Histamine is determined by a
spectrofluorometric assay following a condensation reaction between
histamine and a fluorophore (0-phthaldialdehyde).  The data are
expressed as a percentage of the total available histamine
determined by measuring histamine release following incubation of
cells at $100^{\circ}$ for 5 min in 0.9% NaCl.  The concentration which
significantly increases the histamine release above control levels
is proposed as an index to evaluate the ocular toxicity.

II.  SCIENTIFIC

A.   Endpoint Assay:  Histamine is a important mediator of acute
irritation responses and is responsible for increased vascular
permeability which progresses to edema and allows inflammatory cell
infiltration.  This assay quantitatively measures the release of
histamine from a mixed population of peritoneal cells which should
be related to the ability of a chemical to initiate ocular
irritation.

B.   Correlation with Irritancy Data:  Only three test chemicals
have been evaluated.  Thus, the database is insufficient to fully
evaluate this test in a meaningful manner.

III. ECONOMIC

This test has several drawbacks from a practical point of view.
Test cells must be obtained from live animals and one animal is
required for each test concentration used in a dose-effect study.
Secondly, the analytical procedure requires wet chemistry followed
by a spectrofluorometic analysis.  Thus, this test requires a
higher level technician trained in animal surgery and analytical
chemistry.

IV.  COMMENTS

Although a test of this nature provides additional information not
obtained in cytotoxicity tests, the cells employed must be prepared

from whole animals and the endpoint analysis as currently employed is cumbersome. Recent advances in HPLC analysis of histamine should improve the usefulness of this text.

V.    REFERENCES

Jacaruso, R.B., Barlett, M.A., Carson, S. and Trombetta, L.D. (1985), Release of histamine from rat peritoneal cells in vitro as an index of irritational potential. J. Toxicol. - Cut. Ocular Toxicol. 4:39-48.

D.4.

GROUP:  Inflammation/Immunity

TEST IDENTIFICATION:  Rat Peritoneal Mast Cells/Serotonin Release

I.   LOGISTICAL

   A.   Biological Component:  Rat peritoneal cells obtained from
   female Sprague-Dawley rats.

   B.   Non-biological component:  Standard cell culture techniques
   and supplies.

   C.   Endpoint Assay:  Freshly prepared, mixed population of rat
   peritoneal cells containing 10% mast cells are incubated with $5\text{-}^3H$
   hydroxytryptophan (5-HTP) for 3 h in a water-shaker bath at $37^o$.
   Cells are then washed 3 times by centrifugation (200 xg - 10 min)
   to remove unincorporated 5-HTP and $4.0 \times 10^6$ cells added to 12 x 75
   mm plastic test tubes.  Test chemical is added to the test tubes
   before addition of cells.  Exposure to test chemicals was carried
   out in a water-shaker bath at $37^o$ for 1 min.  Tubes are immediately
   cooled in an ice-water bath and cells pelleted by centrifugation
   (200 xg-5 min at $4^o$).  Supernatants are collected and assayed for
   $^3H$.  Cell pellets are resuspended, boiled for 15 min to release
   remaining $^3H$-label and assayed for $^3H$.  Serotonin release is
   evaluated as a percentage of the total serotonin available for
   release as determined by the heat treatment.

II.   SCIENTIFIC

   A.   Endpoint Assay:  Serotonin release by peritoneal mast cells is
   monitored by prelabeling the cells with 5-HTP which is converted
   intracellularly to serotonin by 5-HTP decarboxylase.  Serotonin is
   a constituent of the basophilic granules in rat mast cells and its
   release reflects stimulation of these cells by chemical toxins.

   B.   Correlation with Irritancy Data:  This test system was
   developed to investigate antiasthmatic changes and as such has not
   been evaluated for its response to ocular toxins.

III.   ECONOMIC

   This is a rapid test involving a 3 h pre-incubation to label cells,
   a 1 min exposure to the test chemical and subsequent radioactivity
   analysis.

IV.   COMMENTS

   This system evaluates the release of an indicator substance by
   mast-cell activation.  Further development may make this approach
   useful for ocular irritation testing.

V.   REFERENCES

Chasin, M.. Scott, C., Shaw, C. and Persico, F. (1979),  A new assay for
the measurement of mediator release from rat peritoneal most cells.
Int. Archs. Allergy Appl. Immun. 58:1-10.

D.5.

GROUP:  Inflammation/Immunity

TEST IDENTIFICATION:   Rat Vaginal Explant/Prostaglandin Release

I.  LOGISTICAL

A.  Biological Component:  Vaginal segments from female Sprague-Dawley rats.

B.  Non-Biological Component:  Standard laboratory supplies.

C.  Endpoint Assay:  Freshly dissected vaginal segments are individually placed in wells of a multi-well tissue culture plate containing 1 ml of Krebs-Ringer bicarbonate buffer, pH 7.0, at room temperature.  This solution serves as an initial rinse.  The tissue segments are next transferred to a treatment well containing test solution and exposed for 30 seconds.  At the end of the exposure period each segment is transferred to another well containing buffer for a post-treatment rinse (approximately 10 seconds).  The tissues are then transferred to fresh medium and incubated at $37^{\circ}$ in a Dubanoff shaking incubator under an atmosphere of 95% $O_2$ / 5% $CO_2$ for 30 min.  After incubation, the buffer is collected and stored at $-70^{\circ}$ until analyzed for prostaglandin $F_{2a}$ and $E_2$ by radioimmunoassay.  The concentration of test chemical which significantly increases prostaglandin release above that of buffer treated controls is considered a positive response.

II.  SCIENTIFIC

A.  Endpoint Assay:  This test system evaluates the release of chemical mediators of inflammation by a physiologically intact mucus membrane.  This approach should be useful for identifying the release of specific initiators of this component of the toxic response.

B.  Correlation with Irritancy Data:  This test system is in a preliminary stage of development and only a limited number of chemicals have been tested.  Additional studies are necessary before this test can be fully evaluated.

III. ECONOMICS

This test requires the preparation of fresh tissues from animals and thus requires technical help familiar with animal surgery. Furthermore, the radioimmunoassay requires radio-detection equipment and appropriate licensing.

IV.  COMMENTS

From a theoretical point of view this test system has potential to provide direct information on the release of chemical mediators of the inflammatory response.  Additional development of the test is required to fully define its potential, however it may be of value to utilize the endpoint assay in test systems which employ biological components more easily acquired and maintained in the laboratory.

V.  REFERENCES

Dubin, N.H., Wolff, M.C., Thomas C.L. and DiBlasi, M.C. (1985), Prostaglandin production by rat vaginal tissue, in vitro response to ethanol, a mild mucosal irritant. Toxicol. Appl. Pharmacol. 78:458-463.

D.6.

GROUP: Inflammation/Immunity

TEST IDENTIFICATION:   Bovine Eye Cup/Histamine (Hm) and Leukotriene C4
                       (LT-C4) Release.

I.   LOGISTICAL

     A.   Biological Component:  Isolated bovine sclerandchoroid
     obtained from a slaughterhouse.

     B.   Non-Biological Component:  The tissues are cultured in Tyrode
     CM buffer in a Dubnoff incubator.

     C.   Endpoint Assay:  Bovine sclerandchoroid complex is obtained by
     removing the ocular adnexa and anterior segment first, then the
     vitreous body and retina with a temporary eversion of the eye.
     Sclerachoroid cups are submerged in Tyrode at $37^\circ$; after 15 min the
     test chemical is added to the culture medium; serial supernatant
     samples are taken for 90 min and immediately derivatized with a
     fluorogenic reagent (Fluorescamine).  Histamine (Hm) and
     leukotriene (LT-C4) are determined by HPLC.  The data are expressed
     as dose-response curves of Hm and LT-C4 release.  The concentration
     which significantly increases Hm and/or LT-C4 release above control
     levels is proposed as an index for the evaluation of ocular
     toxicity.

II.  SCIENTIFIC

     A.   Endpoint Assay:  Histamine and leukotriene C4 are important
     mediators, respectively, of early and late phases of the
     inflammatory response, and both are rapidly released by mast cells.
     This assay quantitatively measures Hm and LT-C4 release from ocular
     tissues, which may be related to chemically induced cell membrane
     damage.

     B.   Correlation with Irritancy Data:  The database not yet
     developed since only four test chemicals have been evaluated.

III. ECONOMIC

     The biological component of the test is relatively inexpensive,
     using eyes from animals sacrificed for other purposes.  The
     preparation of fresh eye tissues requires technical personnel
     trained in animal surgery.  A consideration is that the analytical
     procedure requires HPLC equipment with fluorimetric detection.

IV.  COMMENTS

     This test is rapid (within 1 day) and utilizes a quantitative
     endpoint.  However, availability of freshly enucleated bovine eyes
     relies upon the presence of a slaughterhouse.  An automated HPLC
     system is required to shorten analysis times.

V.   REFERENCES

Benassi, C.A., Angi, M.R., Salvalaio, L. and Bettero, A. (1986),
Histamine and Leukotriene C4 release from isolated bovine sclerachoroid
complex:  a new in vitro ocular irritation test, Chimica oggi
(accepted).

# E.  Recovery/Repair

E.1.

GROUP:  Recovery/Repair

TEST IDENTIFICATION: Rabbit Corneal Epithelial Cells/Wound Healing

I.   LOGISTICAL

A.   Biological Component:  Cultured rabbit primary corneal epithelial cells.

B.   Non-Biological Component:  Standard tissue culture methodologies.

C.   Endpoint Assay: Rabbit corneal epithelial cell cultures are initiated from Dispase II treated corneas of New Zealand white rabbits.  Cultures are established in the absence of a feeder layer in a medium consisting of equal parts of Dulbeccos Modified Eagles Medium and Hams F12 supplemented with 5% fetal bovine serum, cholera toxin (0.1 ug/ml), epidermal growth factor (10 ng/ml), insulin (5 ug/ml), gentamicin (5 ug/ml) and dimethylsulfoxide (0.5% v/v).  Epithelial cells derived from six corneas are pooled and plated into the 6 wells of a 35-mm diameter multiplate.  After 7-10 days, the confluent multilayers are subcultured and the cells derived from each 35-mm diameter well are plated into a 24-well multiplate, each well of which contained 1 ml of the above medium, except that cholera toxin was omitted.  Discs, 6 mm in diameter cut from Millipore HA filters, rinsed in 6 changes of distilled water, boiled in distilled water, and dried in a laminar flow hood prior to use, are placed on the surface of each culture of a 24-well multiplate, gently tapped down, and a stainless steel probe (6 mm in diameter), cooled in liquid nitrogen, is placed against the plastic surface opposite the disc for 5 sec.  The probe is then removed, medium consisting of Dulbeccos Modified Minimal Essential Medium and Hams F12 with the addition of gentamycin and dimethylsulfoxide is added, and the disc carefully lifted out, leaving a discrete circular defect in the cell layer.  Test chemicals are added and cultures are incubated for 42 h.  To determine wound closure, all cultures are drained of medium, fixed with neutral buffered formalin, and stained <u>in situ</u> with full strength Giemsa.  The size of the remaining defect, as revealed by the unstained cell-free area, is determined by projecting the plates onto a screen with an overhead projector at a fixed distance, tracing the unstained area onto paper, and cutting out and weighing the remaining wound area.  The weight was normalized, as a percentage, to that of the initial wound size or converted to area in $mm^2$ for comparison of wound sizes.

II.  SCIENTIFIC

A.   Endpoint Assay:  This test system measures one component of epithelium healing, cell migration, in an objective manner. The lack of a basement membrane in the test system may influence the cellular response observed.

B.    Correlation with Irritancy Data:  Insufficient data are available to make a meaningful evaluation.

III. ECONOMICS

This is a relatively straight forward method.  The test should be comparable in cost to the in vivo rabbit test unless automated, in which case it should cost less per test but instrumentation for video analysis will involve capital investment.  The test protocol takes 3 days to perform if a steady stream of primary cell cultures in wells is available (these take approximately 14 days to develop).

IV.  COMMENT

Test system shows promise as a screening system and can evaluate some components of recovery.  This system has an advantage in that one can establish direct animal/human cell comparisons. It is clear that the system does not evaluate the entire repair process as occurs in vivo but looks at cell migration and adhesion.

V.   REFERENCES

Jumblatt, M.M. and Neufeld, A.H. (1985), A tissue culture model of the human corneal epithelium, In, In Vitro Toxicology A.M. Goldberg (Ed.) Alternative Methods in Toxicology, Vol. 3, Mary Ann Liebert, Inc., New York, 393-404.

Jumblatt, M.M. and Neufeld, A.H. (1986), A tissue culture assay of corneal epithelial wound closure. Invest. Ophthalmol. Vis. Sci. 27:813.

# F. Other

F.1.

GROUP:  Other

TEST IDENTIFICATION:   EYTEX Assay

I.    LOGISTICAL

    A.    Biological Component:  A proprietary mixture of biological
    macromolecules including proteins, glycoproteins and
    mucopolysacharides.

    B.    Non-Biological Component:   Chemical reagents

    C.    Endpoint Assay:  The test procedure consists of two stages.
    The first stage is a qualifying screen to identify the strength of
    reaction and to eliminate materials that interfere with the test
    reaction.  The test chemical is reacted with the test reagent and
    the resulting turbidity compared with that produced by 0.05%
    benzalkonium chloride (BAC).  Depending on the outcome of this test
    a second assay is run with an appropriate series of dilutions to
    determine more accurately the concentration-response relationship.
    The response is measured as concentration of BAC which gives
    equivalent turbidity.  A classification scheme is given in units of
    equivalent BAC concentrations and is divided into seven categories:
    non-irritant, very slight, very mild, mild, low moderate, high
    moderate and severe.

II.   SCIENTIFIC

    A.    Endpoint Assay:  The test system is based on the ability of a
    chemical to produce turbidity in a solution consisting of a mixture
    of biological macromolecules.  Presumably the reaction depends on
    the ability of the test chemical to alter the inter- and
    intra-molecular interactions.  The relationship between the in
    vitro physical-chemical reactions and the mechanism of toxicity of
    chemicals in the eye is unknown, thus, this test must be considered
    purely correlative. Approximately 10-20% of test chemicals
    encountered are incompatible with this test system and cannot be
    evaluated.

    B.    Correlation with Irritancy Data:  For 49 chemicals and
    formulations selected from several chemical classes, the EYTEX
    results correlated well with reported literature values for eye
    irritancy testing.

III.   ECONOMIC

    This is a relatively simple and rapid test which requires little
    technician time.  Calibration, using a spectrophotometer, provides
    quantitation which allows easy interpretation of results.

IV.   COMMENTS

The EYTEX test system is an in vitro test which is based on
turbidity produced in a test tube reaction.  The components of this
system are not identified and thus cannot be evaluated.  This test
requires no animals or tissue culture facilities although the
material is biologically based.  Because of the highly correlative
nature of the test, vigorous evaluation using a large battery of
chemicals in a masked evaluation  protocol is necessary to
determine its potential ability to evaluate eye irritancy.

V. REFERENCES

Gordon, V.C. and Bergmen, H.C. (1986), EYTEX, an in vitro method for
evaluation of optical irritancy.  National Testing Corporation report,
26.

F.2.

GROUP: Other

TEST IDENTIFICATION: Computer Based/Structure Activity Relationship (SAR)

I. LOGISTICAL

A. Biological Component: None - a statistical predictive model.

B. Non-Biological Component: Mainframe or IBM PC computer with proprietary software package.

C. Endpoint Assay: A data set of 1,100 chemicals evaluated in rabbit eye tests and published in the literature are being used to develop an SAR model as follows:

Each chemical is described by means of its features, which can include physico-chemical parameters such as the water/octanol partition coefficient and molar refractivity, as well as substructural parameters describing the substructures of which each chemical is composed. These independent parameters are then used to develop an equation (either regression or discriminant) to model (explain) the variability in the endpoint in terms of the weighted features describing the compounds in the database. Subsequently one can then evaluate how well the endpoints have been modeled. Once a model has been developed it is then possible to take test compounds for which the endpoint has not been measured, develop their features and substitute these into the equation to calculate the probability of the compound having that particular endpoint. In addition to the simple statistical procedures just described, other techniques also are utilized for purposes of identification of nonconforming compounds.

II. SCIENTIFIC

A. Endpoint Assay: A correlative model is highly dependent on the validity of the data which is utilized in developing it. Without a mechanistic basis the regulatory value of such a test system is limited.

B. Correlation with Irritancy Data: The system is currently under development, therefore no predictive data are available.

III. ECONOMIC

Utilization of this test system appears to be highly economical, but specific physical/chemical data concerning the test chemical are required.

IV. COMMENTS

Given the somewhat diverse and poorly characterized nature of the original database from which the model is developed and the lack of any structural/mechanistic basis, the utility of the model is yet to be established. Studies with chemicals not currently included in the database are needed. The treatment of complex mixtures must assume that the effects are additive since there is no theoretical basis for predicting other types of interactions a priori.

V.    REFERENCES

Enslein, K. (1984),   Estimation of toxicology endpoints by
structure-activity relationships, Pharmacol. Rev., 36:131-134.

Enslein, K. and Craig, P.N. (1982),   Carcinogenesis: A predictive
structure activity model, J. Toxicol. Envir. Hlth, 10:521-530.

Enslein, K., Lander, T.R., Tomb, M.E., Landis, W.G. (1983), Mutagenicity
(Ames):  A structure-activity model, J. Teratogenesis, Carcinogen and
Mutagenesis, 3:503-514.

Enslein, K., Tomb, M.E. Lander, T.R. (1984): Structure-activity models
of biological oxygen demand, in QSAR in Environmental Toxicology, Kaiser
KLE, (Ed.), D. Reidel Publishing Co., Dordrecht, Holland.

F.3

GROUP:  Other

TEST IDENTIFICATION:  Tetrahymena/Motility

I.  LOGISTICAL

A.  Biological Component:  The ciliated protozoan <u>Tetrahymena</u> <u>thermophila</u> (available from American Type Culture Collection - ATCC30008).

B.  Non-Biological Component:  Protozoan culture is similar to mammalian cell culture and requires sterile techniques.

C.  Endpoint Assay:  An aliquot of stock culture of $\underline{T}$. <u>thermophila</u> (0.5 ml) is added to 10 ml of MM2 media and incubated at $21^{o}$ for 48 h.  A series of dilutions of test chemical is prepared in MM2 media (1:2, 1:4, ..., 1:32) immediately prior to the test and 50 ul of diluted chemical is mixed with 50 ul of $\underline{T}$. <u>thermophila</u> suspension.  A sample of the mixture is immediately applied to a microscope depression slide and 2 min later examined at 40 or 100 x magnification.  Motility was examined by counting the total number of cells in the sample and the number of cells moving normally. The approximate minimal dillution allowing at least 90% of the cells to move in a relatively normal manner as well as the maximal dilution resulting in at least 90% immotile cells was determined. The reciprocal of these two dilutions was added to determine the test score.  The higher the test score the more irritating the compound.  All tests were performed in triplicate.

II.  SCIENTIFIC

A.  Endpoint Assay:  This assay system evaluates the lethality of test chemicals using a single celled protozoan as the test organism.  The data provided are comparable to the cytotoxicity data obtained using mammalian cells.  The mechanistic relationship between protozoan lethality and ocular irritation is not well defined.

B.  Correlation with Irritancy Data:  Comparative data are reported for 21 test chemicals.  Only a few cases where the test underestimated the severity of test chemicals were noted; however, there were 5 false positives (glycerol, ethylene glycol monoethyl ether, aluminum chlorhydroxide, triethanolamine lauryl sulfate and formaldehyde).

III. ECONOMICS

This is a relatively simple and rapid test based on standard protozoan culture techniques.  Two days are needed to prepare the test organism from stock cultures and only 2 min for exposure and several minutes for counting make this one of the more rapid test protocols.

IV.  COMMENTS

This test is potentially useful as a rapid, prescreen test. However, the fact that protozoans are phylogenetically distant from human ocular tissues raises issues of concern.

V.    REFERENCES

Silverman, J. (1983), Preliminary findings on the use of protozoa
(Tetrahymena thermophila) as models for ocular irritation testing in
rabbits.   Lab. Animal Sci. 33:56-59.

# Chapter 7

# **Validation**

Validation will be defined here to mean the process that the value of new alternative test systems developed from an idea in the research laboratory is assessed for its ability to predict toxicological risk assessment of chemical agents, whether drugs, industrial chemicals or commercial products. The process of validating new in vitro test systems is an essential activity in the sequence of events which will result ultimately in the replacement of eye irritancy testing. To put the validation process in perspective, a short account of the historical development of the Ames assay for evaluating the carcinogenic potential of chemicals is helpful. This test has taken more than 15 years to reach the point where it has been integrated into carcinogenicity testing strategy; during this time, several important lessons were learned which should be kept in mind when validating new alternative test systems for other toxicological endpoints. Some of these can be summarized as follows:

(i) Test Standardization/Technology Transfer: When various laboratories began using the Ames test, it became obvious that slight differences in the test protocol resulted in significant variability in the apparent mutagenic potential of test chemicals. The necessity to rigorously standardize procedural factors (such as time of exposure to test chemicals, culture media composition, preparation of S9 fractions, etc.) in order to obtain reproducible results from one laboratory to the next came to light, a similar lesson was learned from the FRAME validation study; there appears to be a direct relationship between the ability to standardize a test protocol and the ability to transfer that technology to other laboratories.

(ii) "Gold Standard" for Evaluation: Validating testing methodologies for a particular biological endpoint using selected chemicals for which relatively certain knowledge of their effect in the target organism is not known is an inefficient approach to validation. The database for evaluation of the validity of in vitro tests must be accurate and appropriate. In the development of the Ames test, there was uncertainty concerning the actual carcinogenic potential

of some compounds used in the test evaluation; this contributed to
controversy which distracted from the validation process.  A key
factor in any validation program is the development of the "Gold
Standard," i.e., a database for selected chemicals which accurately
describes the specified biological response of interest in the
target population.  As will be discussed below, this is a
particularly difficult problem in eye irritation tests.

(iii) Mechanistic Basis of Test:  An important component in the
acceptance of the Ames test as a useful index of the carcinogenic
potential of chemicals is the rationale that alterations in DNA (as
measured by mutations) contribute to the initiation of cancer in
man.  Although there are limitations to this premise, i.e., other
mechanisms are known to contribute to cancer in man,  this
mechanistic connection allows for a reasonable explanation of
why the test is predictive.  This element of understanding can be
crucial for the acceptance of testing methodologies since it also
allows an explanation of why the test does not work in certain
cases and so provides a basis for defining the limitations of a
particular test.  The greater the ability of a test system to
measure an experimentally defined necessary and sufficient
condition for the development of a particular toxicological
response, the more easily accepted the test will be.

(iv) Limitations of Tests to Certain Chemical Classes:  Clearly, if a
chemical produces its toxic effects through a mechanism not
evaluated by a particular test system, then the predictive powers
of that test for that chemical group will be low.  This statement,
obvious in retrospect, required learning through experience in the
development of the Ames test.  Everyone would like a single test
which would predict toxicity accurately for all possible chemicals
to be tested, but this is highly unlikely.  Hence, a battery of
tests is required with overlapping ranges of validity which when
taken together will provide maximum accuracy in predicting overall
toxicity.

(v)  Historical Precedence/Data Base Development:  Finally, the
acceptance of a new innovative development in biotechnology
requires time to generate a "track record."  Only when new test
systems have been used in several laboratories on an extensive set
of test chemicals will the new technology become accepted and used.
This process takes time.  However, if this stage of test
development is promoted, the time required for the process of
validation can be reduced significantly.

Using the historical perspective gained from the development of the
Ames assay, it is possible to establish an efficient approach to
validation which takes these lessons into consideration and allows the
validation process to proceed at an accelerated rate.  This validation
procedure can be conceptualized as consisting of four phases.

The initial phase of any validation program consists of several
identified steps.  First, it is important to define the objective which
is to be attained by using alternative test systems.  In the case of
ocular irritation, the objective of toxicity testing is to develop a
database which can be utilized to evaluate the potential of chemicals to
produce acute damage to the anterior surface of the eye.  A second
activity is the identification of alternative testing systems which,
when taken together, have the greatest potential to provide the database
necessary for risk evaluation.  This has been defined for ocular
irritation testing and is described in Chapter 5.

TABLE 12.   THE VALIDATION PROCESS

---

PHASE 1:   Preliminaries

        A.   Definition of test objective
        B.   Identification of potential alternative tests
        C.   Selection of test chemicals
        D.   Establishment of "Gold Standard"

PHASE 2:   Microvalidation - Primary Laboratory

        A.   Protocol standardization
        B.   Blind feasibility study (20 test chemicals)

PHASE 3:   Macrovalidation - Secondary Laboratory

        A.   Test implementation - QC samples
        B.   Blind study (50-100 test chemicals)
        C.   Statistical evaluation

PHASE 4:   Test Battery Optimization

---

A third activity in the initial phase is the selection of test chemicals which will be used in blind studies. In fact, two sets of chemicals should be selected. The first set of chemicals would be used in a blind study by the laboratories which have developed specific test systems (designated primary laboratories). This set of approximately 20 chemicals is to be used in the primary laboratory to establish the feasibility of a particular test system. In order for blind studies to be comparable between primary laboratories, a "chemical bank" must be established to provide documented test chemicals for testing, and the testing program must be coordinated by an independent party. The second set of test chemicals, 50-100 in number, is used in the later stages of validation to generate the necessary broad database described below. The criteria used to select both sets of test chemicals should include: (1) a distribution among general toxicity classes (non-irritant, mild irritant, strong irritant, corrosive) which is similar to the distribution expected in the universe of potential test chemicals; (2) a range of chemicals from defined chemical classes to develop structure-activity relationships; (3) some formulations which will provide data concerning mixture interactions; and (4) a minimum set of data relating to the toxicity rating based on eye irritancy testing and the expected human ocular response.

As a final preliminary activity, it is essential to assemble a complete evaluation of the toxicological risk associated with each test chemical selected for the validation study. This set of data, referred to as the "Gold Standard," will be used to evaluate the results of the blind studies. The optimum situation would be to have a set of data which provided a quantitative measure of the toxicological response of the human eye to each chemical using a continuous response scale. In the arena of acute ocular toxicity, such a database does not exist, although qualitative data on human eye damage for some chemicals is available. The result is that value judgments on the "validity" of alternative tests will first have to be based on comparison to Draize eye test rankings. The dilemma created by this situation clearly points out the need for further development of ocular irritation testing. Recent work (Griffith, _et al_., 1980; Freeberg, _et al_., 1984) suggests that the low dose (0.01) eye irritancy protocol is more predictive of human eye response; however, the current database using this protocol is somewhat limited and probably will require additional animal studies to form the basis for validation studies. The potential use of the exfoliative cytology test (Walberg, 1983) and/or the release of mediators of the inflammatory response (for example, histamine - Bettero, et al., 1984) in rabbit eye tests should be investigated. Unfortunately, this also would require significant animal studies to provide an adequate database for validation evaluations. The possibility of human clinical trials to verify the correct classification of non-irritating chemicals would provide useful corroborative data for this particular category of test chemicals.

Having identified the candidate tests, selected the test chemicals and established the "Gold Standard," the next phase (microvalidation) is to develop the new test protocols in the primary laboratories to the point where the specific technology can be transferred to other tester laboratories, referred to as secondary laboratories. This developmental step involves the standardization of the test protocol into a format which can be reasonably expected to provide consistent results when utilized in secondary laboratories. The greater the ability to utilize commercially available products for the test systems, the better the chance of transferring the test technology from primary laboratories to secondary laboratories. It also is important at this phase to run a blind study using approximately 20 chemicals. This study will accomplish two goals. First, it will allow an independent evaluation of the potential value of each test system using known, documented test chemicals. Secondly, the data generated in this blind study will be used for quality control purposes when secondary laboratories set up the new test system. Only when every secondary laboratory can reproduce the results from the primary laboratory on these 20 chemicals will the methodology transfer be considered successful. If such a transfer is not possible, then the test system should be returned to the primary laboratory for further development and standardization. When the technology has been successfully transferred then the final stages of the validation program are ready to proceed.

The third phase (macrovalidation) involves the transfer of the testing technology to the secondary laboratories and the evaluation of this process, using the quality control database established in Phase 2 (microvalidation). The objective of this phase is to determine any technical problems in the implementation of the test protocols in testing laboratories. Following the establishment of the battery of test protocols in a group of secondary laboratories, the next step is to conduct a large scale comparative study employing an extensive collection of test chemicals (50-100). This will provide the necessary database to evaluate fully the potential role of the proposed test in the replacement of the eye irritancy testing as a means of human risk assessment. A statistical analysis of the data generated using the outlook described in Purchase (1982) and recently reviewed in Scala (in press) will provide a useful evaluation of the sensitivity, specificity and predictive value of an individual test system. Assuming that the chemical selection process has chosen test chemicals with a careful consideration for the expected real world distribution of chemicals among the various toxicity classifications, then the predictive value of the test system (as determined in the validation study) will realistically reflect the expected success of the particular test in the commercial testing environment.

A single alternative test is most unlikely to be adequate to evaluate the potential for acute ocular irritation of new chemicals.

Several areas of response are described in Chapter 5 which, although not mutually exclusive, define potential ways of measuring toxic responses: cytotoxicity, cell dysfunction, inflammatory response and repair. A battery of tests for toxicological evaluation should include representative tests of each of these categories to provide a spectrum of data which can be used to generate a toxicological profile.

The exact battery to be used will depend to a certain extent on two factors: (1) the purpose of the testing; and (2) the commercial classification of the chemicals being used. The major purposes of toxicological testing are either to make judgments during product development as to the best candidate among competing chemical structures and formulations or to satisfy defined regulatory requirements for product marketing. In the former case, the strategy for making decisions during product development requires testing, which with minimum effort, will define the best alternatives among the possible choices. This is significantly different from the more complete evaluation necessary for regulatory decisions. The second factor which influences the structure of a test battery is the type of commercial product being tested. As has been discussed in Chapter 3, the testing needs of pharmaceuticals is different from that of industrial chemicals and other classes of commercial products and vice versa. Clearly, a chemical which will be used as an ocular pharmaceutical will require extensive testing for its potential for ocular irritation and, for the foreseeable future, will require animal testing in the final stages. However, commercial chemicals which presumably will only enter the eye by accident need to satisfy labeling requirements where discrimination between non-irritants and mild irritants is not particularly important while strong irritants and corrosives must be clearly defined. The specific battery selected will vary depending on the particular goals of a given institution; and the data generated by the comparative studies in Phase 3 can be used to "tune" the test battery to optimize the testing program for the particular purpose required as well as to minimize cost and time per chemical tested.

With specific reference to the in vitro alternatives to eye irritancy testing, the validation process is still in the identification and development phase ( Phases 1 and 2 ). Some proposed alternative tests have been developed to the point where more than one laboratory has utilized the test protocol on a group of chemicals. Examples where this has occurred are the FRAME and CAM tests. However, in the majority of the proposed tests only the primary laboratory has experience with the test protocol. A preliminary microvalidation study sponsored by the Soap and Detergent Association is currently in progress and results are expected in 1986. Even with this effort, one will not be able to judge the ultimate usefulness of the majority of the proposed test protocols. Until a validation program as described in this chapter is completed, the full potential of alternative approaches to eye irritancy testing will not be realized.

# References

AESECHBACHER, M., C.A. REINHARDT and ZBINDEN, G. (1986), A rapid cell membrane permeability test using fluorescent dyes and flow cytometry. Submitted to Cell Biol. Toxicol.

ALEXANDER, P. (1965), Evaluation of the irritation potential of shampoos and conditioning rinses. specialties. 9:33-37.

ANDERMANN, G. and ERHART, M. (1983), Meth. and Find. Exptl. Clin. Pharmocol. 5:321-333.

BAKER, J.R., (1946), The histochemical recognition of lipine. J. Microsc. Sci 87:441.

BALLANTYNE, B. and SWANSTON, D.W. (1977), The scope and limitations of acute eye irritation tests, Current Approaches in Toxicology, B. Ballantyne (Ed.) John Wright & Sons, Bristol, 139-157.

BALLS, M. and HORNER, S.A. (1985), The FRAME interlaboratory program on in vitro cytotoxicology. Fd. Chem. Toxic., 23:205-213.

BARRITT, G.J. (1981), Calcium transport across cell membranes: progress toward molecular mechanisms. Trends Biochem. Sci. 6:322.

BAUM, J.L., (1963), A histochemical study of corneal respiratory enzymes. Arch. Ophthalmol. 70:103.

BAYARD, S. and HEHIR, R.M. (1976), Evaluation of proposed changes in the modified draize rabbit irritation test. Soc. Toxicol. 15th Meeting, Atlanta, GA. Abstract 225.

BAZAN, N.G. (1984), Effects of ischemia and electroconvulsive shock on free fatty acid pool in the brain. Biochem. Biophys, Acta 218:1.

BAZAN, H.E.P., BICKLE D.L., BEUERMAN, R., BAZAN, N.G. (1985), Cryogenic lesion alters the metabolism of aronchidonic acid in rabbit cornea layers. Invest. Ophthalmol. Vis. Sci. 26:474-480.

BAZAN, E.P., BICKLE, D.L., et. al.(1985), Inflammation-induced stimulation of the synthesis of protaglandins and lipooxygenase-reaction products in rabbit cornea. Current Eye Res. 4:175.

BECKLEY, J.H. (1965), Comparative eye testing: man vs. animal. Tox. App. Pharm. 7:93-101.

BELL, E., SHER, S., HULL, B., MERRILL, C., ROSEN, S., CHAMSON, A., ASSELINEAU, D., DUBERTRET, L., COULOMB, B., LAPPIERE, C., NUSGENS, B. and NEVEUX, Y., (1983), The reconstitution of living skin. J. Invest. Dermatol. 81:2s-10s.

BENASSI, C.A., ANGI, M.R., SALVALAIO, L. and BETTERO, A. (1986), Histamine and Leukotriene C4 release from isolated bovine scheracharoid complex: a new in vitro ocular irritation test, chimica agg; (accepted).

BERGMEYER, H.U. and BERNT, F. (1965), Lactic dehydrogenase. In, Methods of Enzymatic Analysis. H.U. Bergmeyer (Ed.), Academic Press, New York, 736-743.

BERMAN, M., LEARY, R. and GAGE, J. (1980), Evidence for a role of the plasminogen activator-plasmin system in corneal ulceration. Invest. Ophthalmol. Vis. Sci. 19:204.

BERMAN, M. (1980), Collagenase in corneal ulceration. In, Collagenase in Normal and Pathological Connective Tissue, D.E. Woolley and J.M. Evanson (Eds.) J. Wiley and Sons, Chichester.

BERMAN, M., WINTHROP, S., AUSPRUNK, D., ROSE, J., LANGER, R. and GAGE, J. (1982), Plasminogen activator (urokinase) caused vascularization of the cornea. Invest. Ophthalmol. Vis. Sci. 22:191-191.

BERMAN, M., MANSEAU, E., LAW, M. and AIKEN, D. (1983), Ulceration is correlated with degradation of fibrin and fibronectin at the corneal surface. Invest. Ophthalmol. Vis. Sci. 24:1358-1366.

BETTERO, A., ANGI, M.R., MORO, F. and BENASSI, C.A. (1983), Histamine assay in tears by fluorescamine derivatization and high-performance liquid chromatography. J. Chromatography, 310:390-395.

BORENFREUND E. and SHOPSIS, C. (1985), Toxicity monitored with a correlated set of cell culture assays. xenobiotica 15:705-711.

BORENFREUND, E. and BORRERO, O. (1984), In vivo cytotoxicity assays: potential alternatives to the Draize ocular irritancy test. Cell Biol. Toxicol. 1:55.

BORENFREUND E. and PEURNER, J.A. (1984), A simple quantitative procedure using monolayer cultures for cytotoxicity assays (HTD/NR-NE). J. Tissue Culture Methods 9:7-10

BORENFREUND E. and PEURNER, J.A. (1985), Toxicity determined in vitro by morphological alterations and neutral red absorption. Toxicol. Letters, 24:119-124.

BRABEC, R.K., PETERS, B.P., BERNSTEIN, I.A., GRAY, R.H. and GOLDSTEIN, I.J., (1980), Differential lectin binding to cellular membranes in the epidermis of the newborn rat. Proc. Nat. Acad. Sci. U.S.A., 77:477.

BREWITT, H. (1979), Sliding of epithelium in experimental corneal wounds: A scanning electron microscopic study. Acta. Ophthalmol, 57: 945.

BRIDGES, J.W., BENFORD, D.J. and HUBBARD, S.A. (1983), Mechanisms of toxic injury. In, Cellular Systems for Toxicity Testing, C.M. Williams, V.C. Dunkel and V.A. Ray (Eds.). Ann. New York Acad. Sci. 407:42-63.

BUCK, R.C. (1979), Cell migration in repair of mouse corneal epithelium. Invest. Ophthalmol. Vis. Sci., 18:767.

BUEHLER, E.V., NEWMAN, E.A. (1964), A comparison of eye irritation in monkeys and rabbits, Tox. Appl. Pharmacol. 6:701-710.

BURNS, R.P., FORSTER, R.K., et al (1975), Chronic toxicity of local anesthetics on the cornea. In, Symposium on Ocular Therapy, Vol. 10, I. Leopold and R.P. Burns (Eds.), John Wiley and Sons, New York, 31-44.

BURTON, A.B.G., YORK, M. and LAWERENCE, R.S. (1981), The in vitro assessment of severe eye irritants, Fd. Cosmet. Toxicol, 19:471-480.

BYERS, H.R. and FUJIWARA, K. (1983), Stress fibers in situ: immunofluorescence visualization with antiactin, antimyosin and antialpha-actinin. J. Cell Biol., 93:804.

CALABRESE, E.J. (1984), Principles of Animal Extrapolation. John Wiley & Sons, New York. 391-402.

CARPENTER, C.P. and SMYTH, H.F. (1946), Chemical burns of the rabbit cornea. Am. J. Ophthalmol. 29:1363-1372.

CHAN, K.Y. and HASCHKE, R.H. (1981), Action of a trophic factor(s) from rabbit corneal epithelial culture on dissociated trigeminal neurons. J. Neurosci. 1:1155.

CHAN, K.Y. and HASCHKE, R.H. (1983),: Isolation and culture of coreal cells and their interactions with dissociated trigeminal neurons. Exp. Eye Res. 35:137.

CHAN, K.Y., (1985), An in vitro alternative to the Draize test. In In Vitro Toxicology. A.M. Goldberg (Ed.), Alternative Methods In Toxicology, Vol. 3, Mary Ann Liebert, Inc., New York 405-422.

CHAN, P.K., HAYES, A.W. (1985), Assessment of chemically induced ocular toxicity; A survey of methods. Toxicology of the Eye, Ear and Other Special Senses A.W. Hayes. (Ed.) Raven Press, New York. 103-143.

CHANG, J., LIU, M.C. and NEWCOMBE, D.S. (1982), Amer. Rev. Resp. Dis., 126:457-459.

CHASIN, M., SCOTT, C., SHAW, C. and PERSICO, F. (1979), A new assay for the measurement of mediator release from rat peritoneal most cells. Int. Archs. Allergy Appl. Immun./ 58:1-10.

CHIFFELLE, T.L. and PUTT, F.A., (1951), Propylene and ethylene glycol as solvents for sudan IV and sudan black B. Stain Technol, 26:51.

CLARK, G., (1979), Displacement. Stain Technol, 54:111.

CLARK, G., (1981), Miscellaneous Methods. In, Staining Procedures, G. Clark (Ed.), 4th Ed., Williams & Wilkins, Baltimore, 206-207.

CRISSMAN, H.A., DARZYBRIEWICZ, Z., TOBEY, R.A. and STEINKAMP, J.A. (1985), Correlated measurements of DNA, RNA and protein in individual cells by flow cytometry. Science 228:1321-1323.

CODE OF FEDERAL REGULATIONS, Revised Jan 1, 1981, Title 16: Subchapter C - Federal Hazardous Substances Act, Part 1500.42, 1981, (Test for Eye Irritants).

CPSC (1976), Illustrated Guide For Grading Eye Irritation Caused By Hazardous Substances. 16 CFR 1500.

DABELSTEEN, E. VEDTOFTE, P., HAKOMORI, S.I. and YOUNG, W.W. (1982), Carbohydrate chains specific for blood group antigens in differentiation of human oral epithelium. J. Invest. Dermatol 79:3-7.

DANNENBERG, A.M. JR., MEYER, O.T., ESTERLY, J.R. and KA,BARA, T. (1968), The local nature of immunity in tuberculosis, illustrated histochemically in dermal BCG Lesions. J. Immunol. 100:931-941.

DORAN, T.I., VIDRICH, A., SUN, T.T. (1980), Intrinsic and extrinsic regulation of the differentiation of skin corneal and esophageal epithelial cells. Cell 22:17-25.

DOUGLAS, H.J. and SPILLMAN, S.D. (1983), In vitro ocular irritancy testing. In, Product Safety Evaluation, A.M. Goldberg (Ed.), Alternative Methods in Toxicology, Vol. 1, Mary Ann Liebert Inc., New York, 205-230.

DRAIZE, J.H., WOODARD, G., CALVERY, H.O. (1944), Methods for the study of irritation and toxicity of substances applied topically to the skin and mucus membranes, J. Pharmacol. Exp. Ther. 82:377-390.

DUBIN, N.H., DE BLASI, M.C., et al (1984), Development of an in vitro test for cytotoxicity in vaginal tissue: effect of ethanol on prostanoid release. In, Acute Toxicity Testing: Alternative Approaches, A.M. Goldberg (Ed.), Alternative Methods In Toxicology, Vol 2., Mary Ann Liebert, Inc., New York, 127-138.

DUBIN, N.H. (1985), Prostaglandin production as an index of in vitro cytotoxicity. In, In Vitro Toxicology, A.M. Goldberg (Ed.), Alternatives Methods In Toxicology, Vol. 3, Mary Ann Liebert, Inc., New York, 43-52.

DUBIN, N.H. WOLFF, M.C., THOMAS, C.L. and DiBLASI, M.C. (1985), Prostaglandin production by rat vaginal tissue, in vitro, response to ethanol, a mild mucosal irritant. Toxicol. Appl. Pharmacol. 78:458-463.

DUNCAN, J.L., (1974), Characteristics of streptolysin O hemolysis: kinetics of hemoglobin and 86 rubidium release. Infect. Immunity, 9:1022.

DUNKEL, V.C. (1983), Biological significance of end points. In, Cellular Systems for Toxicity Testing, G.M. Williams, V.C. Nunbrel and V.A. Ray (Eds.), New York Acad. Sci. 407:43-41.

DUNN, B.J., NICHOLS, C.W. and GAD, S.C. (1982), Acute dermal toxicity of two quarternary organophosphonium salts in the rabbit. Toxicology 24:245-250.

ELGEBALY, S.A., FOROUHAR, F., GILLIES, C., WILLIAMS, S., O'ROURKE, J. and KRUETZER, D.L. (1984), Neovascularization of the cornea: current concepts of its pathogenesis. Am. J. Path. 116:407-416.

ELGEBALY, S.A., GILLIES, C., FOROUHAR, F., HASHEM, M., BADDOUR, M., O'ROURKE, J. and KRUETZER, D.L. (1985), An in vitro model of leukocyte mediated injury to corneal epithelium. Current Eye Res., 4:31.

ELGEBALY, S.A., NABAWI, K., HERKBERT, N., O'ROURKE, J. and KRUETZER, D.L. (1985), Characterization of neutrophil and monocyte specific chemotactic factors derived from the cornea in response to injury. Invest. Ophthalmol. Vis. Sci., 26:320.

ELGEBALY, S.A., HERKERT, N., O'ROURKE, J. and KRUETZER, D.L. (1986), Characterization of neutrophil and monocyte specific chemotactic factors derival from the cornea in response to hydrogen peroxide injury. Submitted for publication.

ELGEBALY, S.A., DOWNES, R.T.. FOROUHAR, F., O'ROURKE, J. and KREUTZER, D.L. (1986), Inflammatory mediators in alkali - burned corneas: Inhibitory effects of citric acid. Submitted for publication.

ELIASON, J., DESHMUKH, A. and ELLIOTT, J.P. (1984), Chemotactic Activity from the corneal epithelium. Invest. Ophthalmol. Vis. Sci. Arvo Abstracts, 25:323.

ENSLEIN, K. and CRAIG, P.N. (1982), Carcinogenesis: a prediction structure activity model, J. Toxicol. Envir. Hlth., 10:521-530.

ENSLEIN, K., LANDER, T.R., TOMB, M.E. and LANDIS, W.G. (1983), Mutagenicity (Ames): a structure-activity model, J. Teratogenesis, carcinogenesis and mutagenesis, 3:503-514.

ENSLEIN, K. (1984), Estimation of toxicology endpoints by structure-activity relationships, Pharmacol. Rev., 36:131-134.

ENSLEIN, K., TOMB, M.E. and LANDER, T.R. (1984), Structure-activity models of biological oxygen demand, In, QSAR in Environmental Toxicology, Kaiser KLE, (Ed.), D. Reidel Publishing Co., Dordrecht, Holland.

EPA (1979), Acute Toxicity Testing Criteria for New Chemical Substances, EPA 560/13-79-009, 9-14.

ETZLER, M.E. and BRANSTRATOR, M.L. (1974), Differential localization of cell surface and secretory components in rat intestinal epithelium by use of lectins. J. Cell Biol. 62:29.

EVANS. W.H. (1977), In, Laboratory Techniques in Biochemistry and Molecular Biology, T.S. Work and E. Work (Eds.). Vol. 7, North Holland, New York, 1-266.

FALAHEE, K.J., ROSE, C.S., SEIFRIED, H.F. and SAWHNEY, D. (1982), Alternatives in toxicity testing. In, Product Safety Evaluation A.M. Goldberg (Ed.) Alternative Methods in Toxicology, Vol. 1, Mary Ann Liebert, Inc., New York, 137-162.

FALAHEE, K.J., ROSE, C.S., OLIN, S.S. and SEIFRIED, H.E. (1981), Eye Irritation Testing: An Assessment of Methods and Guidelines for Testing Materials for Eye Irritancy Office of Pesticides and Toxic Substances, EPA, Washington, D.C.

FDA (1965) Illustrated Guide for Grading Eye Irritation by Hazardous Substances, Washington, DC.

Federal Hazardous Substances Act (1964), File 21.CFR 13009-191.12. Test for Eye Irritants. Federal Register.

FORBES. I.J. (1963), Studies of cytotoxicity using 32p. Austral. J. Exp. Biol, 41:255.

FRANKE, W.W., APPELHAUS, B., SCHMID, E., FREUDENSTEIN, C., OSBORN, M. and WEBER, K. (1979), Identification and characterization of epithelial cells in mammalian tissue by immunofluorescence microscopy using antibodies to prekeratin. Differentiation, 15:7-25.

FRANKE, W.W., SCHILLER, D.L., MOLL, R., WINTER, S., SCHMID, E. and ENGELBRECHT, I. (1981), Diversity of cytokeratins: differentiation-specific expression of cytokeratin polypeptides in epithelial cells and tissues. J. Molec. Biol, 153:933-959.

FRAZIER, J.M. (1985), Specific protein synthesis as an indicator of cellular injury. In, In Vitro Toxicology, A.M. Goldberg (Ed.), Alternative Methods In Toxicology, Vol. 3, Mary Ann Liebert, Inc. New York, 189-198.

FREEBERG, F.E., GRIFFITH, J.F., BRUCE, R.D. and BAY, P.H.S. (1984), Correlation of animal test methods with human experience for household products. J. Toxicol.- Cut Ocular Toxicol. 1:53-64.

FRIEDENWALD, J.S., HUGHES, W.F. and HERRMANN, H. (1944), Archives of Ophthalmology, 31:279.

FRIEND, J., KINOSHITA, S., THOFT, R.A. and ELIASON, J.A. (1982), Corneal epithlial cell cultures on stromal carriers. Invest. Ophthalmol. Vis. Sci, 23:41-49.

FROMER, C.H. and KLINTWORTH, G.K. (1976), An evaluation of the role of leukocytes in the pathogenesis of experimentally induced corneal vascularization: III. Studies related to the vasoproliferation capability of polymorphonuclear leukocytes and lymphocytes. Am. J. Path, 82:157.

FUCHS, E. and GREEN H. (1980), Changes in keratin gen expression during terminal differentiation of the keratinocyte. Cell, 19:1033.

GAD, S.C. WALSH, R.D. and DUNN, B.J. (1986), Correlation of ocular and dermal irritancy of industrial chemicals. J. Toxicol.- Cut. and Ocular Toxicol, 5:3,193-211.

GALE, E.F. (1974), The release of potassium ions from Candida albicans in the presence of polyene antibiotics. J. Gen. Microbiol. 80:451.

GALLIN, J.I. and QUIE, P.G. (1978), Leukocyte Chemotaxis: Methods Physiology and Clinical Implications. Raven Press, New York.

GILMAN, M.R. (1982), Skin and eye testing in animals. Principles and Methods of Toxicology A.W. Hayes, (Ed.) Raven Press, New York, 209-222.

GILMAN, M.R., JACKSON, E.M., CERVEN, D.R. and MORENO, M.T. (1983), Relationship between the primary dermal irritation index and ocular irritation. J. Toxicol.- Cut and Ocular Toxicol, 2:107-117.

GIPSON, I.K. and ANDERSON, R.A. (1977), Actin filaments in normal and migrating corneal epithelial cells. Invest. Ophthalmol. Vis. Sci., 16:161.

GIPSON, I.K. and ANDERSON, R.A. (1980), Effect of lectins on mirgration of the corneal epithelium. Invest. Ophthalmol. Vis. Sci., 22:633.

GIPSON, I.K., AND KIORPES, T.C.(1980), Effects of tunicamycin on migration of corneal epithlium. Eur. J. Cell Biol. 22:361a.

GIPSON, I.K., WESTCOTT, M.J. and BROOKS, N.G. (1982), Effects of cytochalasins B and D and colchicine on migration of the corneal epithelium. Invest. Ophthamol. Vis. Sci., 22:633-642.

GIPSON, I.K. and KEEZER, L. (1982), Effects of cytochalsins and colchicine on the ultrastructure of migrating corneal epithelium. Invest. Ophthalmol. Vis. Sci., 22:643.

GIPSON, I.K. and KIORPES, T.C. (1982), Epithelial sheet movement: protein and glycoprotein synthesis. Dev. Biol., 92:259.

GLOXHUBER, C.H. (1985), Modification of the draize eye test for the safety testing of cosmetics, Fd. Chem. Toxic, 23:187-188.

GOLDMAN, R.D., SCHLOSS, J.A. et al (1976), Organizational changes of actinlike microfilaments during animal cell movement. In, Cell Motility, R. Golman, T. Pollard and J. Rosenbaum (Eds.) Cold Spring Harbor Laboratory, New York, 27-247.

GORDON, V.C. and BERGMEN, H.C. (1986), EYTEX, an in vitro method for evaluation of optical irritancy. National Testing Corporation report, 26.

GOSPODAROWICZ, D. and TUBER, J.P. (1980), Growth factors and extracellular matrix. Endocrine. Rev., 1:201.

GRABNER, G., SINZINGER, H., LUGER, T.A., HUBEY-SPITZY, V. and STUR, M. (1984), A corneal epithelial system sytokine (CETAF) stimulates prostaglandin production by corneal fibroblast, Invest. Ophthalmol. Vis. Sci., Arvo Abstracts, 258:299.

GREEN, W.R., SULLIVAN, J.B., HEHIR, R.M., SCHARPF, L.F. and DICKINSON, A.W. (1978), A systematic Comparison of Chemically Induced Eye Injury in the Albino Rabbit and the Rhesus Monkey. The Soap and Detergent Association, New York.

GRIFFITH, J.F., NIXON, G.A., BRUCE, R.D., REER, P.J. and BANNAN, E.A. (1980), Dose-response studies with chemical irritants in the albino rabbit eye as a basis for selecting optimum testing conditions for predicting hazard to the human eye. Tox. Appl. Pharmacol. 55:501-513.

GRISSMAN, H.A., DARZYBRIEWICZ, Z., TOBEY, R.A. and STEINKAMP, J.A. (1985), Correlated measurements of DNA, RNA and protein in individual cells by flow cytometry. Science, 228:1321-1323.

GUILLOT, J.P., GONNET, J.F., CLEMENT, C., CAILLARD, L. and TRAHAUT, R. (1982), Evaluation of the cutaneous-irritation potential of 56 compounds, Fd. Chem. Toxic. 201:563-572.

GUILLOT, J.P., GONNET, J.F., CLEMENT, C., CAILLARD, L. and TRUHAUT, R. (1982), Evaluation of the ocular-irritation potential of 56 compounds, Fd. Chem. Toxicol. 20:573-582.

HAIK, B.C. and ZIMMY, M.L. (1977), Scanning electron microscopy of corneal wound healing in the rabbit. Invest. Ophthalmol. Vis. Sci, 16:787.

HAWKES, S.P. and BARTHOLOMEW, J.C. (1977), Quantitative determination of transformed cells in a mixed population of simultaneous fluorescence analysis of cell surface and DNA in individual cells. Proc. Natl. Acad. Sci. U.S.A., 74:1626.

HAY, E.D. (1978), Fine structure of embryodic matrices and their relation to the cell surface in Ruthenium red-fixed tissues, Growth 42:399-423.

HENDERSON, D. and WEBER, K. (1979), Three-dimensional organization of microfilaments and microtubules in the cytoskeleton. Exp. Cell Res., 124:301.

HENDRIX, M.J.C., HAY, E.D., MARK, K.V.D. and LINSENMAYER, T.F. (1982), Immunohistochemical localization of collagen types I and II in the developing chick cornea and tibia by electron microscopy. Invest. Ophthalmol. Vis Sci. 22:359-375.

HENNEY, C.S. (1973), Studies on the mechanism of lymphocyte mediated cytolysis. The use of various target cell markers to study cytolytic events. J. Immunol., 110:73.

HINGSON, D.J., MASSENGILL, R.K. and MAYER, M.M. (1969), The kinetics of release of 86Rubidium and hemoglobin from erythrocytes damaged by antibody and complement. Immunochem. 6:295-307.

HIRST, L.W., KENYON, K.R., FOGLE, J.A., HANNINEN, L. and SPARK, W.J. (1981), Comparative studies of cornea surface injury in the monkey and rabbit. Arch. Ophthalmol., 99:1066-1073.

HOCHOCHKA, P.W. (1986), Defense strategies against hypoxia and hypothermia. Science, 231:234.

HOLMES, R.P., MAHFOUZ, M., TRAVIS, B.D., YOSS, N.L. and KEENAN, M.J. (1983), The effect of membrane lipid composition on the permeability of membranes to Cadmium In, Biomembranes and Cell Functions, F.A. Kummerov, G. Benga and R.P. Holmes (eds.), Ann. New York Acad, Sci., 414:44-56.

HORISBERGER, M. AND ROSSET, J. (1977), Colloidal gold, a useful marker for transmission and scanning electron microscopy. J. Histochem. Cytochem., 25:295.

HSIE, A.W., SCHENLEY, R.L., TAN, E.L., PERDUE, S.W., WILLIAMS, M.W., HAYDEN, T.L. and TURNER, J.E. (1984), The toxicity of sixteen metallic compounds in Chinese hamster ovary cells: a comparison with mice and drosophila. In, Acute Toxicity Testing: Alternative Approaches, A.M. Goldberg (Ed.), Alternatives Methods In Toxicology, Vol. 2, Mary Ann Liebert, Inc. New York, 115-126.

HULL, D.S., RILEY, M.V., CSUKAS, S. and GREEN, K. (1982), Corneal endothelial glutathione after photo-dynamic change. Invest. Ophthalmol. Vis. Sci., 22:405-408.

INTERAGENCY REGULATORY LIAISON GROUPS (January 1981), Testing Standards and Guidelines Work Group. Recommended Guidelines.

JACARUSO, R.B., BARLETT, M.A., CARSON, S. and TROMBETTA, L.D. (1985), Release of histamine from rat peritoneal cells in vitro as an index of irritational potential, J. Toxicol.-Cut. Ocular Toxicol. 4:39-48.

JACKSON, E.M. (1983), Industrial Practices in Safety Testing. In, Product Safety Evaluation, A.M. Goldberg (Ed.), Alternative Methods in Toxicology, Vol. 1, Mary Ann Liebert, Inc., New York, 51-65.

JACKSON, J. and RUTTY, D.A. (1985), Ocular tolerance assessment-integrated tier policy, Fd. Chem. Toxic, 23:309-310.

JACOBUS, W.E. and MOREADITH, R.W. (1983), Control of heart oxidative phosphorylation by creatine kinase in mitochondrial membranes. In, Biomembranes and Cell Function, F.A. Kummerov, G. Benga and R.P. Holmes (Eds.). Ann. New York Acad. Sci., 414:73-89.

JESTER, J.V., RODRIQUES, M.M. and SUN, T.T. (1985), Change in epithelial keratin expression during healing of rabbit corneal wounds. Invest. Ophthalmol. Vis. Sci., 26:828-837.

JUMBLATT, M.M., FOGLE, J.A. and NEUFELD, A.H. (1980), Cholera toxin stimulates adenosine 3'5'-monophosphate synthesis and epithelial wound closure in the rabbit cornea. Invest. Ophthalmol. 19:1321-1327.

JUMBLATT, M.M. and NEUFELD, A.H. (1981), Characterization of cyclic AMP-mediated wound closure of the rabbit corneal epithelium. Curr. Eye Res. 1:189.

JUMBLATT, M.M. and NEUFELD, A.H. (1985), A tissue culture model of the human corneal epithelium. In, In Vitro Toxicology, A.M. Goldberg (Ed.), Alternatives Methods In Toxicology, Vol. 3, Mary Ann Liebert, Inc., New York, 391-404.

JUMBLATT, M.M. and NEUFELD, A.H. (1986), A tissue culture assay of corneal epithelial wound closure. Invest. Ophthalmol. Vis. Sci. 27:813.

KASTEN, F.H. (1981), Acridine dyes. In, Encyclopedia of Microscopy and Microtechnique, P. Gray (Ed.), Rheinhold, New York, 4-7.

KASTEN, F.H., BURTEN, V. and GLOVER, P. (1959), Flourescent Schiff-type reagents for cytochemical detection of polyaldehyde moieties in sections and smears. Nature,. 184:1797-1798.

KAUFMAN, H.E. and KATZ, J.I. (1976), Endothelial damage from intraocular lens insertion. Invest. Ophthalmol., 15:996.

KELLER, H.U. and TILL, G.O. (1983), Leukocyte Locomotion and Chemotaxis, Birkhauser Verlag Basel, Stuttgart.

KEMP, R.V., MEREDITH, R.W.J., GAMBLE, S. and FROST, M. (1983), A rapid cell culture technique for assaying to toxicity of detergent based products in vitro as a possible screen for high irritants in vivo. Cytobios, 36:153-159.

KEMP R.V., MEREDITH, R.W.J. and GAMBLE, S. (1985), Toxicity of commercial products on cells in suspension: A possible screen for the Draize eye irritation test. Fd. Chem. Toxic., 23:267-270.

KENYON, K.R. (1969), The synthesis of basement membrane by the corneal epithelium in bullous keratopathy. Invest. Ophthalmol., 8:156.

KENYON, K.R., FOGLE, J.A., STONE, D.L. and STARK, W.J. (1977), Regeneration of corneal epithelial basement membrane following thermal cauterization. Invest. Ophthalmol. Vis. Sci., 16:292-301.

KLEIN, G. and PEILMANN, P. (1963), In vitro cytotoxic effect of isoantibody measured as isotype release from labelled target cell DNA. Nature, 199:451.

KLINTWORTH, G.K. (1973), The hamster cheek pouch: An experimental model of corneal vascularization. Am. J. Path. 73:691.

KLINTWORTH, G.K. and BURGER, P.C. (1983), Leukocyte-mediated injury to corneal endothelial cells: A model of tissue injury. Intl. Ophth. Clinc. 23:27.

KLYCE, S.D. and CROSSON, C.E. (1985), Transport processes across the rabbit corneal epithelium: a review. Current Eye Res., 4:323.

KNOX, P., UPHILL, P.F., FRY, J.R., BENFORD, D.J. and BALLS, M. (1986), The FRAME multicent project on in vitro cytotoxicity. Fd. Chem. Toxic. (in Press).

KOETER, H.B.W.M. and PRINSEN, M.K. (1985), Introduction of an in vitro eye irritation test as a possible contribution to the reduction of the number of animals in toxicity testing. CIVO Institutes TNO Report No. V85.188/140322.

KULKARNI, P.S. and SRIVIVASIN, B.D. (1981), The effect of topical and intraperitoneal indomethacin on the generation of PGE 2-like acitivity in rabbit conjunctiva and iris ciliary body. Exp. Eye Res., 33:121.

KUWABARA, T., PERKINS, D.G. and COGAN, D.G. (1976), Sliding of the epithelium in experimental corneal wounds. Invest. Ophthalmol., 15:4-14.

LANTZ, E., DYSTER-AAS, K., et al (1978), In Vitro release of fibrinolytic activators from cornea. Albrecht v. Graefes Arch. Klin. Exp. Ophthalmol., 206:157.

LATVEN, A.R. and MOLITOR, H., (1939), Comparison of the toxic, hypnotic and irritating properties of 8 organic solvents, J. Pharm. Exptl. Ther: 65,89-94

LAZARIDES, E. and WEBER, K. (1974), Actin antibody: the specific visualization of actin filaments in non-muscle cells. Proc. Natl. Acad. Sci. U.S.A., 71:2268.

LAWRENCE, R.S., GROOM, M.H. ACKROYD, D.M. and PARISH, W.E. (1986), The chorioallantoic membrane in irritation testing. In Press, Food Chem. Toxicol.

LEIGHTON J., TCHAO, R., VERDONE, J. and NASSAUER, J. (1985), Macroscopic assay of focal injury in the chorioallantoic membrane. In, In Vitro Toxicology, A.M. Goldberg (Ed.), Alternatives Methods In Toxicology, Vol. 3, Mary Ann Liebert. Inc., New York., 355-370.

LEIGHTON, J., NASSAUER, J. and TCHAO. R. (1985), The chick embro in toxicology: An alternative to the rabbit eye. Fd. Chem. Toxic., 23:291-298.

LEIGHTON, J., NASSAUER, J. TCHAO, R. and VERDONE, J. (1983), Development of a procedure using the chick egg as an alternative to the Draize rabbit test. In, Product Safety Evaluation, A.M. Goldberg (Ed.), Alternative Methods in Toxicology, Vol. 1, Mary Ann Liebert, Inc., New York, 165-177.

LEOPOLD, I.H. (1982), Pharmacology of cellular elements of inflammation. In, Biomedical Foundations of Ophthalmology, I.H. Leopold (Ed.), Vol. 3, Harper and Row Publ. Inc., New York, 33.

LUEPKE, N.P. (1985), Hen's egg chorioallantoic membrane test for irritation potential, Fd. Chem. Toxic., 23:287-291

LEUPKE, N.P. (1985), HEP-Chorionallantois-test: an alternative to the Draize Rabbit Eye Test. In, In Vitro Toxicology To Animal Testing, A.M. Goldberg (Ed), Alternatives Methods In Toxicology, Vol. 3, Mary Ann Liebert, Inc., New York, 591-606.

LILLIE, R.D. (1956), A nile blue staining technique for the differentiation of melanin and lipofuscins. Stain Technol., 31:151.

LILLIE R.D. and FULLMER, H.M. (1976), Histopathologic Technic And Practical Histochemistry. Ed. 4, McGraw-Hill, New York.

LUJDA, Z. and GROSSRAN, R. (1979), Glucose-6-phosphate dehydrogenase. In, Enzyme Histochemistry., Springer-Verlag, Berlin, 282-284.

MacCORNAILL, M.A. and GURR, E. (June 1964), The histological properties of rhondonile blue. Irish J. Med. Sci., 6th Ser. Nos. 457-468, 243-250.

MacGREGOR, II, R.D. and TOBIAS, C.A. (1972), Molecular sieving of red cell membranes during gradual osmotic hemolysis. J. Memb. Biol. 10:345.

MADOFF, M.A., ARTENSTEIN, M.S. and WEINSTEIN, L. (1963), Studies in the biological activity of purified staphylococcal alpha-toxin. II. The effect of alpha-toxin on Ehrlich oscities carcinoma cells. Yale J. Biol. Med. 35:382-389.

MADOFF, M.A., COOPER, L.Z. and WEINSTEIN, L. (1964), Hemolysis of rabbit erythrocytes by purified staphylococcal alpha-toxin. III. Potassium release. J. Bacteriol. 87:145-149.

MANN, I. and PULLINGER, B.D. (1942), A study of mustard gas lesions of the eyes of rabbits and men, Proc. R. Soc. Med. 35:229-244.

MARTZ, E., BURAKOFF, S.J. and BENACERRAF, B. (1974), Interruption of the sequential release of small and large molecules from tumor cells by low temperature during cytolysis mediated by immune T-cells or complement. Proc. Natl. acad. Sci. U.S.A., 71:177-181.

MARZULLI, F.N. and RUGGLES, D.I. (1973), Rabbit Eye Irritation Test: Collaborative Study, J. Assoc. Off. Anal. Chem., 56:905-914.

MAURICE, D.M. (1985), Pain and Acute Toxicity Testing in the Eye. In, In Vitro Toxicology, A.M. Goldberg (Ed.), Alternative Methods in Toxicology, Volume 3, Mary Ann Liebert, Inc., New York.

MAYER, B.W., JR., HAY, E.D. and HYNES, R.O. (1981), Immunocytochemical localization of fibronectin in embryonic chick trunk and area vesculosa. Dev. Biol., 82:267-286.

McCALLY, A.W.; FARMER, A.G. and LOOMIS, E.C. (1933), Corneal ulceration following use of lash lure, JAMA 101:1560-1561.

McCORMICK, J.F. NASSAUER, J., BIELUNAS, J. and LEIGHTON, J. (1984), Anatomy of the chick charioallantoic membrane relevant to its use as a substrate. in bioassay systems. Scanning Electron Microscopy IV, 2023-2030.

McDONALD, T.O., SEABAUGH, V., SHADDUCK, J.A. and EDELHAUSER, H.F. (1983), Eye Irritation., Dermatotoxicology. F.N. Marzulli and H.I. Maibach (Eds.) Hemisphere Publishing, New York. 555-610.

McLAUGHLIN, R.S. (1946), Chemical burns of the human cornea. Am. J. Ophthalmol. 29:1355-1362.

THE MERCK MANUAL OF DIAGNOSIS AND THERAPY (1982), R. Berkaw (Ed.), Merck, Sharp & Dome Res. Labs. 14th edition.

MOWRY, R.W. (1975), Special value of prestaining polyanions with basic dyes of contrasting color (alcian blue) before staining with aldehyde fuchsin with particular reference to pancreatic islet B cells and the diagnosis of mesidoblastosis. J. Histochem. Cytochem., 23:322.

MUIR, C.K., FLOWER, C. and VAN ABBE, N.J. (1983), A novel approach to the search for in vitro alternatives to in vivo eye irritancy testing. Toxicol. Let., 18:1-5

MUIR, C.K. (1983), The toxic effect of some industrial chemicals on rabbit ileum in vitro compared with eye irritancy in vivo. Toxicol. Let. 19:309-312.

MUIR, C.K. (1984), Asimple method to assess surfactant-induced bovine corneal opacity in vitro: Preliminary findings. Toxicol. Let. 23:199-203.

MUIR, C.K. (1985), Opacity of bovine cornea in vitro induced by surfactants and industrial chemicals composed with ocular irritancy in vivo. Toxicol. Let. 24:157-162.

MULLER, B.J. and GROSS, J. (1978), Regulation of corneal collagenase production: Epithelial-stromal cell interactions. Proc. Natl. Acad. Sci. U.S.A., 75:4417.

MURPHY, J.C., OSTERBERG, R.E., SEABAUGH, V.M. and BIERBOWER (1982), Ocular irritancy response to various pHs of acids and bases with and without irrigation. Toxicology 23:281-291.

NAMBA, M., DANNENBERG, A.M., JR. and TANAKA, F. (1983), Improvement of the histochemical demonstration of acid phosphatase, B-galactosidase and nonspecific esterase in glycol methcrylate tissue sections by cold temperature embedding. Stain Technol. 58:207-213.

NAS (1977), Principles and Procedures for Evaluating the Toxicity of Household Substances, NAS Publication 1138, 41-59.

NG, M.C. and RILY, M.V. (1980), Relation of intracellular levels and redox state of glutathione to endothelial function in the rabbit cornea. Exp. Eye Res., 30:511.

NORK, T.M., HOLLY, F.J., HAYES, J., WENTLANDT, T. and LAMBERTS, D.W. (1984), Timolol inhibits corneal epithelial wound healing in rabbits and monkeys. Arch. Ophthalmol. 102:1224-1228.

NORTH-ROOT, H., YACKOVICH, DEMETRULIAS, F.J. GUCULA, N. and HEINZE, J.E. (1982), Evaluation of an in vitro cell toxicity test using rabbit corneal cells to predict the eye irritation potential of surfactants. Toxicol. Letters., 14:207-212.

NORTH-ROOT, H., YACKOVICH, F., DEMETRULIAS, J., GUCULA, N. and HEINZE, J.E. (1985), Prediction of the eye irritation potential of shampoos using the in vitro SIRC toxicity test. Fd. Chem. Toxic., 23:271-273.

OLIVER, G.J.A. and PEMBERTON, N.A. (1985), An in vitro epidermal slice technique for identifying chemicals with potential for severe cuganeous effects. Fd. Chem. Toxic., 23:229-232.

PANDOLFI, M. and LANTZ, E. (1979), Parital purification and characterization of keratokinase, the fibrinolytic activator of the cornea. Exp. Eye Res., 29:563.

PFISTER, R.R. (1975), The healing of corneal epithelial abrasions in the rabbit: a scanning electdron microscope study. Invest. Ophthalmol. 14:648.

POPPER, H. (1941), Histologic distribution of vitamin A in human organs under normal and pathologic conditions. Arch. Pathol. 31:766.

PRICE, J.B., BARRY, M.P. and ANDREWS, I.J. (1986), The use of chick chorioallantoic membrane to predict eye irritants. In Press. Food Chem. Toxicol.

PRICE, J.B. and ANDREWS, I.J. (1985), The in vitro assessment of eye irritation using isolated eye. Fd. Chem. Toxic, 23:313-480.

PROSAD, S.P. and MUKHERJEE, C. (1983), Metabolic activation of adipocytes by insulin accompanied by an early increase in intracellular pH. In, Biomembranes and Cell Function, F.A. Kummerov, G. Benga and R.P. Holmes (Eds.), Ann. New York Acad Sci, 414:347-351.

PRUNERIERAS, M., REGINIER, M. and WOODLEY, D. (1983), Methods for cultivation of keratinocytes with an air-liquik interface. J. Invest. Dermato. 81:Suppl No. 1, 28s-33s.

PURCHASE, I.F.H. (1982), ICPEMC Working Paper 2/An appraisal of predictive tests for carcinogenicity. Mutation Research, 99:53-71.

REINHARDT, C.A. and SCHLATTER, CH. (1985), Acute irritation tests in risk assessment, Fd. Chem. Toxic. 23:145-148.

REINHARDT, C.A., PELLI, D.A. and ZBINDEN, G. (1985), Interpretation of cell toxicity data for the estimation of potential irritation. Fd. Chem. Toxic., 23:247-252.

RILEY, M.V. and YATES, E.M. (1977), Glutathione in the epithelium and endothelium of bovine and rabbit cornea. Exp. Eye Res. 25:385.

RILEY, M.W. (1985), Pump and leak in regulation of fluid transport in rabbit cornea. Current Eye Res., 4:371.

ROBBINS, E., MARCUS, P.I. and GONATAS, N.K. (1964), Dynamics of acridine orange-cell interaction; II. Dye-induced ultrastructural changes in multivesicular bodies (acridine orange particles.) J. Cell Biol., 21:49.

ROTMAN, B. and PAPERMASTER, B.W. (1966), Membrane properties of living mammalian cells as studied by enzymatic hydeolysis of fluorogenic esters. Proc. Natl. Acad. Sci, U.S.A., 55:134.

ROUZER, C.A., SCOTT, W.A., GRIFFITH, O.W., HAMILL, A.L. and COHN, Z.A. (1981), Depletion of glutathione selectively inhibits synthesis of leukotriene C by marophages. Proc. Natl. Acad. Sci. U.S.A., 78:2532-2536.

ROUZER, C.A., SCOTT W.A., GRIFFITH, O.W., HAMILL, A.L. and COHN, Z.A. (1982), Arachidonic acid metabolism in glutathione deficient macrophages. Proc. Natl. Acad. Sci. U.S.A., 79:1621-1625.

ROWLAND, F.N., DONOVAN, M.J., LINDSAY, M., WEISS, W.I., O'ROURKE, J. and KREUTZER, D.L. (1983), Demonstration of inflammatory mediator-induced inflammation and endothelial cell damage in the anterior segment of the eye. Am. J. Path., 110:1-12.

SAARNI, H. and TAMMI, M. (1978), Time and concentration dependence of the action of cortisol on fibroblasts in vitro. Biochem Biophys. Acti, 540:117.

SAUNDERS, A.M. (1964), Histochemical indentification of acid mucopolysaccharides wih acridine orange. J. Histochem. Cytochem., 12:164.

SCAIFE, M.C. (1982), An investigation of detergent action on in vitro and possible correlations with in vivo data. Internat. J. Cosm. Sci. 4:179-193.

SCAIFE, M.C. (1985), An in vitro cytotoxicity test to predict the ocular irritation potential of detergents and detergent products. Fd. Chem. Toxic., 23:253-258.

SCALA, R.A., (In Press), Theoretical approaches to validation in: In Vitro Toxicology - Approaches to Validation. A.M. Goldberg (Ed.), Alternative Methods in Toxicology, Vol. 5, Mary Ann Liebert, Inc., New York.

SCHLESINGER, M.J. and ASHBURNER, M. AND TISSIERAS, A. (Eds.) (1982), Heat Shock: From Bacteria to Man. Cold Spring Harbor Laboratory, New York.

SCHWARTZ, B.D. and McCULLEY, J.P. (1981), Morphology of transplanted corneal endothelium drived from tissue culture. Invest. Ophthalmol. Vis. Sci., 201:467.

SELLING, J. and EKWALL, B. (1985), Screening for eye irritancy using cultured Hela cells. Xenobiotica, 15:713-717.

SHADDUCK, J.A., EVERITT, J. and BAY, P. (1985), Use of in vitro cytotoxicity to rank ocular irritation of six surfactants. In, In Vitro Toxicology. Goldberg (Ed.) Alternative Methods in Toxicology, Vol. 3, A. Mary Ann Liebert, Inc., New York, 641-649.

SHADDUCK, J.P., RENDER, J., EVERITT, J., MECCOLI, R.A. and ESSEX-SORLIE, D. (In Press), An approach to validation: comparison of six materials in three tests. In, In Vitro Toxicology - Approaches to Validation, Alternative Methods in Toxicology, Vol. 5, Mary Ann Liebert, Inc., N.Y.

SHOPSIS, C. and BORENFREUND, E. (1985), In vitro cytotoxicity assays: potential alternatives to the Draize test. In, Evaluation Des Effects Cosmetiques Methodes D'Aumourd'Hai et de Demain, proceedings of Xvemes Journees Internationales de Dermocosmetologie de Lyon, June 5, 6, 7, 1985.

SHOPSIS, C., BORENFREUND, E., WALBERG, J. and STARK, D.M. (1984), In vitro cytotoxicity assays as potential alternatives to the Draize ocular irritancy test. In, Acute Toxicity Testing: Alternative Approaches, A.M. Goldberg (Ed.), Alternative Methods In Toxicology, Vol. 2. Mary Ann Liebert, Inc., New York, 101-114.

SHOPSIS, C. and SATHE, S. (1984), Uridine uptake inhibition as a cytotoxicity test: Correlation with the Draize test. Toxicology 29: 195-206.

SHOPSIS, C. (1984), Inhibition of uridine uptake and cultured cells: A rapid, sublethal cytotoxicity test. J. Tissue Culture Methods 9:19-22.

SHOPSIS, C., BORENFREUND, E., WALBERG, J. and STARK, D.M. (1985), A battery of potential alternatives to the Draize test: uridine uptake inhibition, morphological cytotoxicity, macrophage chemotaxis and exfoliative cytology. Fd. Chem. Toxic., 23:259-266.

SHOPSIS, C. and ENG, B. (1985), Uridine uptake and cell growth cytotoxicity tests: comparison, applications and mechanistic studies. J. Cell Biol. 101:87a.

SHOPSIS, C. and ENG, B. (1986), Modulation of in vitro cytotoxicity assessments by serum and solvents. In vitro, In press.

SHOPSIS, C. and ENG. B. (1985), Rapid cytotoxicity testing using a semi-automated protein determination on cultured cells. Toxicol. Letters., 26:1-8.

SILVERMAN, J. (1983), Preliminary findings on the use of protozoa (Tetrahymena thermophila) as models for ocular irritation testing in rabbits. Lab. Animal Sci., 33:56-59.

SIMONS, P.J. (1981), An alternative to the Draize test. In, The Use of Alternatives in Drug Research, A.N. Rowan and C.J. Stratmann (Eds.), The MacMillan Press Ltd., London.

SOONG, H.K. and CITRON, C. (1985), Different corneal epithelial healing mechanisms in rat and rabbit: role of actin and calmodulin, Invest. Ophthalmol. Vis. Sci., 26:838.

STARK, D.M., SHOPSIS, C., BORENFREUND, E. and WALBERG, J. (1983), Alternative approaches to the Draize assay: chemotaxis, cytology, differentiation and membrane transport studies. In, Product Safety Evaluation, A.M. Goldberg (Ed.), Alternative Methods in Toxicology, Vol. 1, Mary Ann Liebart, Inc., New York, 179-204.

SUGRUE, S. and HAY, E.D. (1981), Response of basal epithelial cell surface and cytoskeleton to solubilized extracellular matrix molecules. J. Cell Biol., 91:45.

SUGRUE, S. and HAY, E.D. (1982), Interaction of embryonic corneal epithelium with exogenous collagen, larminin and fibronectin: Role of endogenous matrix molecules. Dev. Biol., 92:97.

SUN, T.T. and GREEN, H. (1976), Differentiation of the epidermal keratinocyte in cell culture: formation of the cornified envelope. Cell 9:511.

SUN, T.T. and GREEN, H. (1977), Cultured epithelial cells of cornea, conjunctiva and skin: absence of marked intrinsic divergence of their differentiated states. Nature, 269:489.

SUN, T.T. and GREEN, H. (1978), Immunofluorescent staining of keratin fibers in cultured cells. Cell, 14:469.

SUN, T.T. and SHIH, C. and GREEN, H. (1979), Keratin cytoskeletons in epithelial cells of internal organs. Proc. Natl. Acad. Sci. U.S.A., 76:2813-2817.

SUNDAR-RAJ, C.V., FREEMAN, I.L. and BROWN, S.I. (1980), Selective growth of rabbit corneal epithelial cells in culture and basement membrane systhesis. Invest. Ophthalmol. Vis. Sci., 19:1222-1230.

SWANSTON, D.W. (1985), Assessment of the validity of animal techniques in eye irritation testing, Fd. Chem. Toxic, 23:169-173.

TAKAHASHI, N., (1982), Cytotoxicity of mercurial preservatives in cell culture. Ophthalmic Res., 14:63.

TAYLOR R.F., PRICE. T.H., SCHWARTZ, S.M. and DALE, D.C. (1981), Neutrophil-endothelial cell interactions on endothelial monolayers grown on milipore filters. J. Clin. Invest., 67:584-587.

THELESTAM, M and MOLLBY, R. (1975), Determination of toxin-induced leakage of different size nucleotides through the plasma membrane of human diploid fiberblast. Infect. Immunity, 11:640.

THELESTAM, M. and MOLLBY, R. (1975), Sensitive assay for detection of toxin-induced damage to the cytoplasmic membrane of human diploid fibroblasts. Infect. Immunity, 12:225.

THELESTAM, M. and MOLLBY, R. (1976), Cytotoxic effects on the plasma membrane of human diploid fibroblasts - a comparative study of leakage test. Medical Biol., 54:39.

THELESTAM, M. and MOLLBY, R. (1979), Classification of microbial, plant and animal cytolysins based on their membrane effects on human fibroblasts. Biochem. Biophys. Acta, 557:156.

TOOLE, B.P. (1976), Binding and precipitation of soluble collagens by chick embroy cartilage proteoglycan. J. Biol. Chem., 251:895.

TRESLSTAD, R.L., HAYASHI, K. and TOOLE, B.P. (1974), Macromolecular order and morphogenesis in basement membrane. J. Cell Biol., 62:815-830.

TRUMP, B.F., BEREZESKY, I.K. and OSORNIO-VARGAS, A.R. (1981), In, Cell Death In Biology and Pathology, I.D. Bowen and R.A. Lockshin (Eds.), Chapman and Hall, London, 209-242.

VAES, G. (1980), I. Cellular secretion and tissue breakdown: cell to cell interactions in the secretion of enzymes of connective tissue breaksown, collagenase and proteoglycan-degrading neutral proteases. A review. Agents and Actions, 10:474.

VAN BUSKIRK, E.M. (1979), Corneal anesthesia after timolol maleate therapy. Am. J. Ophthalmol, 88:739.

VAN BUSKIRK, E.M. (1980), Adverse rections from timolol afministration. Ophthalmology, 87:477.

WALBERG, J. (1983), Exfoliative cytology as a refinement of the Draize eye irritancy test. Toxicol. Lett., 18:49.

WALKER, A.P. (1985), A more realistic animal technique for predicting Human Eye Responses, Fd. Chem. Toxic., 23:175-178.

WALUM, E. (1982), Membrane lesions in cultures mouse neuroblastoma cells exposed to metal compounds. Toxicology, 25:67.

WEHLAND, J., OSBORN, M. and WEBER, K. (1979), Cell to substrate contacts in living cells. a direct correlation between interference reflexion and indirect immunofluorescence microscopy using antibodies against actin and alpha-actinin. J. Cell Sci., 37:257.

WEIL, C.S. and SCALA, R.A. (1971), Study of intra- and interlaboratory variability in the results of rabbit eye and skin irritation tests, Tox. Appl. Pharmacol., 19:276-360.

WEISSMAN, G. (1980), Prostaglandins in acute inflammation. Current Concepts, The Upjohn Co.

WEST, D.C., HAMPTON, I.N., ARNOLD, F. and KUMAR, S. (1985), Angiogenesis induced by degradation products of hyaluronic acid. Science, 228:1324-1326.

WHIKEHART, D.R. and EDELHAUSER, H.F. (1978), Glutathione in rabbit corneal endothelial: the effects of selected perfusion fluids. Invest. Ophthalmol. Vis. Sci., 17:455.

WIGZELL, H. (1965), Quantitative titrations of mouse H-2 antibodies using 51 CR-labelled target cells. Transplantation, 3:423.

WILKINSON, P.C. (1982), Chemotaxis and Inflammation, 2nd Ed., Churchill Livingston, London.

WILLIAMS, S.J., GRAEPEL, G.J. and KENNEDY, G.L. (1982) Evaluation of ocular irritancy potential: intralaboratory variability and effect of dosage volume. Toxicol. Letters, 12:235-241.

WILLIAMS, S.J. (1984), Prediction of ocular irritancy potential from dermal irritation test results, Fd. Chem. Toxic., 2:157-161.

WILLIAMS, S.J. (1985), Changing concepts of ocular irritation evaluation: pitfalls and progress, Fd. Chem. Toxic., 23:189-193.

WILLIAMS, T. (1959), Detoxification Mechanisms, Chapman and Hall, London.

# A Critical Evaluation of Alternatives to Acute Ocular Irritation Testing